The essential guide to
health care for adults with Down syndrome

Vee Prasher | Anisha Prasher

British Library Cataloguing in Publication Data

A CIP record for this book is available from the Public Library

© BILD Publications 2014

BILD Publications is the imprint of:
British Institute of Learning Disabilities
Birmingham Research Park
97 Vincent Drive
Edgbaston
Birmingham B15 2SQ

Telephone: 0121 415 6960

E-mail: enquiries@bild.org.uk

Website: www.bild.org.uk

No part of this book may be reproduced without prior permission from the publisher, except for the quotation of brief passages for review, teaching or reference purposes, when an acknowledgement of the source must be given.

ISBN 978 1 905218 30 1

BILD Publications are distributed by:
BookSource
50 Cambuslang Road
Cambuslang
Glasgow G32 8NB

Telephone: 0845 370 0067

Fax: 0845 370 0068

For a publications catalogue with details of all BILD books and journals e-mail enquiries@bild.org.uk or visit the BILD website www.bild.org.uk

Printed in the UK by Latimer Trend and Company Ltd, Plymouth

People with learning disabilities and people with autism want to make their own choices and decisions about the things that affect their lives. To help make this happen, BILD works to influence policy-makers and campaigns for change, and our services can help organisations improve their service design and develop their staff to deliver great support.

Contents

Dedication		4
About the authors		5
Acknowledgements		5
Preface		6
Introduction		8

Personal and social issues

Chapter 1	Intellectual and social development	18
Chapter 2	Growth and nutrition	21
Chapter 3	Health professionals and support services	28

Specific medical issues

Chapter 4	Vision and related issues	38
Chapter 5	Hearing and related issues	47
Chapter 6	Heart and circulation	53
Chapter 7	Respiratory system	64
Chapter 8	Digestive system	73
Chapter 9	Sexual health	85
Chapter 10	Urinary system	97
Chapter 11	Nervous system	102
Chapter 12	Skeleton, joints and dental care	109
Chapter 13	Skin conditions	119
Chapter 14	Hormonal and blood-related issues	125
Chapter 15	Psychological, emotional and mental health issues	137

Appendices and resources

Appendix A	Glossary of additional medical terms	150
Appendix B	Medical checklist	151
Appendix C	IQ tests	154
Appendix D	Further reading and sources of information	156
Appendix E	Details of organisations and websites for further information and advice	160
Appendix F	Index	164

Dedication

This book is dedicated to Beryl Smith BSc, Dip Ed. Psych., PhD. Beryl was a co-author with Professor Vee Prasher of the textbook *Down Syndrome and Health Care* published in 2002. Beryl worked in the field of learning disability for over 30 years, as an educational psychologist, researcher, teacher trainer and university lecturer. During the 1990s she set up a master's course for professionals working with adults with a learning disability in the community. After retirement she was the editor of *The SLD Experience*, a journal published by BILD for parents and practitioners working with and caring for children and young people with severe and profound learning difficulties. After a short illness she sadly died in 2011 but her contribution to the field of intellectual disability is very much appreciated.

About the authors

Vee P Prasher MB, ChB, MMedSc, MRCPsych, MD, PhD, F.IASSID
Professor Vee Prasher is a Professor of Neuropsychiatry and Consultant Psychiatrist in Birmingham, UK. He has an internationally recognised reputation in the field of Down syndrome, having published over 150 articles and published seven textbooks on many aspects of physical and psychological issues in adults with Down syndrome. He has completed several post-doctorate degrees (MMedSc, MD, PhD) highlighting important health issues for people with Down syndrome. Professor Prasher has clinical responsibility for a large number of adults with learning disabilities in the West Midlands with ongoing teaching and research responsibilities. He works as a medical advisor to the Down's Syndrome Association in the UK. He is involved in a number of international research studies investigating the causes, treatment and prevention of Alzheimer's disease in adults with Down syndrome.

Anisha Prasher BMBS BMedSci
Dr Anisha Prasher is a medical doctor working in both primary and secondary care in the East Midlands, UK. She completed her BMedSci and BMBS at Nottingham University. Since qualifying she has worked in both adult and paediatric settings, with an interest in general medicine and health care for people with Down syndrome. She is at present undertaking a number of research projects into the genetics of ill-health in adults with Down syndrome.

Acknowledgements

Our thanks to all the individuals with Down syndrome, their families and numerous professionals in the West Midlands, who allowed us to spend time with them to collect information for this book.

Preface

This book, a revised version of the textbook *Down Syndrome and Health Care* has been written to promote better understanding of the health care needs of adults with Down syndrome. Many books are already available giving general information to families of children with Down syndrome, with more specialised medical textbooks available to clinicians and academics regarding disorders in adults with the syndrome.

There is, however, a need for a book giving straightforward, practical information on aspects of health that an adult with Down syndrome may experience during his or her lifetime. This book aims to meet that need.

Most adults with Down syndrome live in the community and it is vital that individuals themselves, family members and paid staff are aware of the health issues that can occur. Professionals in the health service are not always fully aware of the health care needs of people with a learning disability and this situation needs to be addressed. The up-to-date and practical information presented in this book will be of help to professionals, family members and paid staff. It deals with both minor and more serious health conditions, their possible causes and how they can be prevented and treated. It aims to improve awareness of the most important physical and psychological issues encountered among adults with Down syndrome.

The book does not aim to give detailed medical information on all aspects of health in adults with Down syndrome. Rather, it gives an overview of the most common and important health issues faced by people with Down syndrome, professionals, family members and paid staff. The book cannot replace a medical assessment, but aims to improve care for adults with Down syndrome by suggesting that, in cooperation with the individual, family members or paid staff can manage minor concerns and alert health care professionals to more serious problems. It will also help readers understand more about the medical procedures and treatments people are likely to experience for more serious conditions and therefore be in a better position to support an adult with Down syndrome.

This book is divided into three parts. The first part *Personal and Social Issues* discusses general issues relating to good health for adults with Down syndrome. The second part *Specific Medical Issues* focuses on health issues in defined areas. The third part *Appendices and Resources* gives details about other sources of support and information.

By turning to a particular chapter, readers can find information on the most significant conditions associated with that area of health. From the index of everyday terms, readers can be guided to the relevant condition.

Introduction

Adults with Down syndrome are now living longer than previously, many into their 60s and 70s. During the 20th century, the average life-expectancy increased progressively: from an estimated 9 years in 1929 to 12 years in 1947, then to 18 years by 1961, 30 years by 1973 and 57 years at the start of the 21st century. In the Western world 80% of children born recently with Down syndrome are expected to survive to the age of 5 years, 72% to the age of 30 years, 44% to the age of 60 years and 14% to 68 years.

With no significant fall in the birth rate of babies with Down syndrome (around one in every 1,000 births) and with adults with Down syndrome living longer, people with Down syndrome will, during the next few decades, become a significant proportion of the population. In the UK, from 2007 to 2008, 1,843 cases of Down syndrome were diagnosed during pregnancy, and 743 babies were born with the condition. Down syndrome affects all ethnic groups equally. Boys are slightly more likely to be born with Down syndrome than girls. No specific cause or causes of Down syndrome have been identified, but the biggest risk factor for the condition is the age at which a woman gives birth. The older a woman is when she has a baby, the higher the risk. The greatest risk (1 in 30) is associated with women who are 45 years of age or over.

It is predicted that the number of people with Down syndrome in the UK will continue to rise, from over 26,000 in 1981 to over 27,000 in 2021. Between 1990 and 2010 the number of people with Down syndrome older than 40 years is thought to have increased by about 75%, but the number of those aged 50 years or more is likely to have risen by about 200%. Such figures are likely to be an under-estimate, as many people with Down syndrome are not known to services. These findings demonstrate a slow but steady rise in the population of people with Down syndrome, for whom health remains an important matter.

Health care for adults with Down syndrome
Adults with Down syndrome are susceptible to the same range of medical problems as the general population, but are also more likely to experience the following particular ailments:

- heart problems
- increased risk of hearing and vision loss
- thyroid disease
- skin problems
- obesity
- memory loss in older adults

Lack of appropriate medical care can dramatically affect quality of life for all of us and can also have a significant impact on the wellbeing of those close to us. The prevention and treatment of health concerns are of considerable importance, not only medically, but also educationally, emotionally, psychologically and socially. Like everyone else in the population, people with Down syndrome are entitled to high quality health care which enables them to achieve healthy and fulfilling lives.

Targeting health care for adults with Down syndrome
Until relatively recently, many adults with Down syndrome were either supported by their families or lived in large institutions. Over the past 30 years, however, the move to care in the community for people with a learning disability has meant that most adults with Down syndrome are now living in the community. Many live with their families, others in their own home with support, or in statutory, voluntary or private residential accommodation. These changes mean that high quality mainstream health care through the local GP surgery is essential.

Responsibility for health care provision

Current policies state that people with a learning disability should access mainstream health care services. This particularly applies to primary health care providers such as general practitioners (GPs) who have an increasing number of patients with a learning disability. However, GPs are often unaware of how many people with Down syndrome are on their lists and are unfamiliar with their associated physical and psychological conditions and the different agencies involved in providing support.

Annual health checks for adults with Down syndrome still need to be more widely implemented. Regular health checks from the GP, community nurse, optician, dentist, audiologist and other health care professionals as required are important for the person to stay healthy (see Appendix B). There remains, therefore, a considerable degree of unmet need.

For some people with Down syndrome there is the additional situation that family members or paid staff may not recognise the symptoms of ill-health or else consider them to be inevitably associated with the syndrome. Good health care may be difficult to access because of transport problems, conventional appointment systems and waiting rooms which are not necessarily suitable for people with learning disabilities and, most importantly, the challenges of communication between the person with a learning disability and the health care professional involved.

Health action plans
Increasingly, we are all becoming more responsible for our own health. Many adults with Down syndrome have the capacity to make decisions regarding their health, providing they have the right support. Information and advice for people with Down syndrome on how to prevent and better manage their own health needs remains an area for future development, although there is an increasing amount of support available, as shown in the appendices and also by an internet search. One approach which can help is the use of a health action plan.

A health action plan is a personal plan about what a person with Down syndrome needs to do to stay healthy. It lists any help and support they may need. Information about the person's health is written down in the health action plan and they can, if they wish, share it with the people supporting them, or just keep it for personal use.

A health action plan has several benefits:

- It allows a person to control their own health
- It helps them to share information about their health with others if they wish – for example a nurse, dentist, doctor etc
- It helps them make sure they have all the health checks they need to stay healthy
- It helps them communicate with others about how they are feeling
- It enables them to learn more about their health and what they need to do to keep well, such as eating healthy foods or doing more exercise

You can find examples of different types of health action plans at www.easyhealth.org.uk.

What is a Health Passport?

As well, or sometimes instead of, a health action plan, many people with a learning disability now have their own health passport. The format and content of a health passport can vary in different parts of the country. Some are comprehensive and cover all aspects of the person's health such as details of their GP and other health professionals, emergency arrangements, medication and existing health conditions, allergies, equipment used, communication needs etc.

Alternatively, in some areas, people with a learning disability may have a hospital passport to take with them when they go for outpatient or inpatient treatment. The hospital passport is for the nursing and medical staff to read. It usually covers things the medical professionals need to know such as the person's name, age, address, GP details, next of kin and religion, existing medical conditions and medication. It should also include details about how the person communicates and their support needs while in hospital. One section might include details about things that are important to the person such as how others would know they are in pain, personal care needs, food requirements, sleeping needs etc. Finally a hospital passport might include details about the person's likes and dislikes.

The role of family members and paid staff

As for all of us, health care for a person with Down syndrome begins at birth, and possibly before birth. People with Down syndrome, their family members and paid staff need to be alert to any medical complications that can occur at any stage of life. High quality health care provision based on prevention and early detection is essential for a good quality of life.

Following the passing of The Mental Capacity Act 2005 legislation in England and Wales there is a duty on all statutory and non-statutory organisations to take into account the views of family members and paid staff when health decisions need to be made with a person with learning disabilities. This is particularly important if it is assessed that the person lacks capacity to make a decision themselves. Family members and paid staff who know a person well have an important role to play in supporting and enabling them to understand any treatment that is proposed, or to be involved in 'best interest' decisions. In Scotland, the Adults with Incapacity Act (Scotland) 2000 provides a similar framework to safeguard the welfare and support of people who lack capacity due to a mental disorder or inability to communicate. In Northern Ireland there is currently no legislation covering advocacy for people who lack capacity.

Different levels of health care support

The level of health care support required by adults with Down syndrome can vary from routine screening to more immediate acute care. The following short stories illustrate this:

Stella
Stella is a 26-year-old woman who has Down syndrome. She lives with her mother in their home close to the city centre. Although Stella went to a school for children with special needs she left at 18 to work part-time in a nearby superstore. In the evenings she attends college and helps in a local youth centre. She is physically fit and well, needing only to wear glasses for short-sightedness. She maintains a healthy weight by dieting and regular exercise. Stella says, 'Mum laughs when I put my video on and jump up and down.' Stella is able to read and write well, catch the bus to work on her own and is proud to admit, 'It's not mum who looks after me; it's me who looks after mum.' She thinks about having a boyfriend but says, 'I've not met the right man yet!' She is taking no prescribed medication but is seen once a year by her doctor for a routine health check.

The complex needs of a person with Down syndrome are highlighted by the following story.

John

At the age of 48, John, a man with Down syndrome, was living in the family home with his mother aged 79 years. He had two sisters, both married with their own children and living away from home. John saw them on his birthday and at Christmas time. He enjoyed playing with his nephews and nieces.

When John was born his mother was told by the hospital staff, 'There's nothing we can do for you. Your son is a 'mongol' and will not live very long. You're better off putting him into an institution and getting on with your life...' John's mother ignored the advice and provided care and support for John with little or no contact with health or social services. At 47, John was rushed to accident and emergency at the local hospital following what turned out to be a seizure.

John recovered and went home. His GP subsequently referred him to a consultant psychiatrist in learning disabilities. On assessment it was found that John had fallen down the stairs six months earlier and was refusing to go upstairs again. He preferred to sleep on the couch downstairs. He had become housebound, refusing to leave the house or even walk in the garden. He was less able than a year previously, requiring more and more help from his mother to dress, wash, feed and walk. He appeared to be unhappy and would scream for no apparent reason. He had lost weight and at times was irritable towards his mother. Blood and urine tests revealed untreated hypothyroidism and a urinary tract infection. John made some improvement with thyroxine hormone replacement therapy and a course of antibiotics for the infection. During the next two months John had two further seizures, became confused, showed evidence of impaired memory and was diagnosed as having Alzheimer's disease - a form of dementia common in adults with Down syndrome.

His mother continued to provide care and initially refused to accept any support. She experienced ill health herself. After several care reviews at home she accepted home care support three days a week and community nurse support twice a week. Following further changes in his needs John had to be transferred to a nursing home. His mother received ongoing support throughout this difficult time.

Unlike Stella, John has more complex health needs. His story demonstrates the importance of information for family members, paid staff and professionals on the physical, psychological, social and family issues relating to the health of all adults with Down syndrome. It may also be necessary to have a more comprehensive and sustained specialist investigation to discover what exactly the problem is.

Robert's story, which follows, highlights the role of annual health checks, health action plans and nursing support.

Robert
Robert is a 36 year old man with Down syndrome who lives in a group home and visits his GP for his annual health check. Three years ago he had a health action plan developed with his GP as he had a number of health concerns. He had become forgetful, put on weight, was less interested in his hobbies, had reduced his exercise activities, spent most of his time at home, and was more irritable. As part of the health investigations he was found by the GP to have hypothyroidism and was prescribed thyroxine replacement therapy. During the subsequent months there was a good response; he became more active, began to participate in sport, lost his excess weight, and was much happier again. In his health action plan it was proposed that he should have routine blood tests for his thyroid status every year that should be facilitated by the community nurse. At his most recent visit to the health centre his thyroid function tests showed that

he had hyperthyroidism; too much thyroxine hormone was circulating in his body. His prescribed thyroxine dosage was reduced. If he had not had his routine annual health check facilitated by his community nurse this may not have been detected.

Robert, with the support from the community learning disability nurse, developed his own health passport so that he could show it to all of the doctors and other professionals he was in contact with so that they were aware of his thyroid disorder and prescribed medication, and the need for him to have routine blood tests. His thyroxine blood levels can be too high or too low and subsequently affect his mental and physical wellbeing.

Robert's story highlights the important role of annual health checks, health action plans and the support from community health care workers such as the GP and community nurse.

Personal and social issues

Chapter 1

Intellectual and social development

The intellectual and social development of children and adults with Down syndrome was in the past generally neglected and ignored. Caring for people with Down syndrome used to be largely based on a medical model of care which made the assumption that Down syndrome was not a curable condition and therefore there was little emphasis placed on supporting the person to develop educationally and socially.

Since the 1950s a more person centred and rights based approach to supporting people with a learning disability has developed based on a social model of disability. It is now accepted that access to education is a human right and that intervention and stimulation can improve the level of both intellectual development and social competence or 'adaptive behaviour'. Adaptive behaviour is defined in terms of self-direction, responsibility and socialisation. Adaptive behaviour includes the age-appropriate behaviours needed by a person to live independently and to keep safe, encompassing such real life skills as dressing, staying safe in the community, food preparation, the ability to work, managing money, making friends and social skills.

This holistic approach to supporting a person is an important factor in their development and growth as an equal and valued citizen in our society.

Intellectual functioning

The concept of the Intelligence Quotient (IQ) has had a considerable impact in defining level of intellectual ability. It can be calculated by using psychological tests such as The Wechsler Adult Intelligence Scale (Revised), but results may be influenced by factors such as life experiences, the degree of cooperation, dexterity and anxiety of the person being tested. This makes accuracy uncertain, particularly for a person with a learning disability. Skilled use of appropriate IQ tests can be used to define the severity of a learning disability, but nowadays what a person can do in terms of self-care and social skills is also considered important and is incorporated into defining the level of ability.

Currently, assessments of how people can manage with their daily living skills (known as their adaptive function), are considered more useful in assessing the impact of any learning disability on a person, than a test of intelligence or

IQ. Adaptive function tests tend only to be used when an assessment is required for a specific purpose and are therefore not generally available for every person with a learning disability. What someone can achieve doesn't necessarily relate to their IQ score, as it depends on the opportunities they have had to learn the skills needed for everyday life and social interaction.

IQ tests are no longer routinely used because their value and use is questioned by many professionals. However, intelligence testing using IQ tests which produce a numerical score are still accepted in some medical, educational and legal settings as the basis for confirming a diagnosis of learning disabilities. Appendix C includes more information about IQ tests.

The level of intellectual functioning for adults with Down syndrome is largely determined by their ability level as a child. The benefit of early intervention programmes for children with Down syndrome remains controversial but some researchers argue that such programmes can have a significant impact on the improvement of both intellectual and social skills. The possible benefits of nutritional supplementation on early intellectual and social development are discussed in Chapter 2.

Despite the fact that in adults the level of intellectual functioning is less liable to change than in children, individuals of all ages and abilities have the potential to learn new things throughout their life. With good support it is possible for many people with Down syndrome to live independently with the right support, have happy and fulfilled lives, work and enjoy friendships and personal relationships.

Social competence
Social competence is a general term used to describe an individual's ability with respect to their degree of independence, level of self-care, ability to be responsible and interact appropriately with others. Most adults with Down syndrome can dress and undress themselves but some need support or prompting. At 21 years of age, approximately two-thirds of adults with Down syndrome are fully independent in toileting (day and night), and half in bathing and dressing. Nearly all adults with Down syndrome have good mobility with the vast majority able to participate in a number of sports. However, some of the characteristics associated with Down syndrome, such as obesity or heart disease, can limit a person's capacity to enjoy some sports activities.

Adults with Down syndrome can learn the usual self-care and personal skills, but may do so at a slower pace than others. A small minority with severe or profound learning disability may require significant support. However, social competence continues to improve with increasing age from adolescence into early adulthood. After this age there is a plateau effect up to the age of 40-50 years when middle-aged adults with Down syndrome can begin to lose skills, eg in mobility, toileting skills, eating and personal care (see figure 1). This may reflect 'premature ageing' or decline associated with the onset of dementia (Chapter 15).

Figure 1 **Level of social competence at different ages**

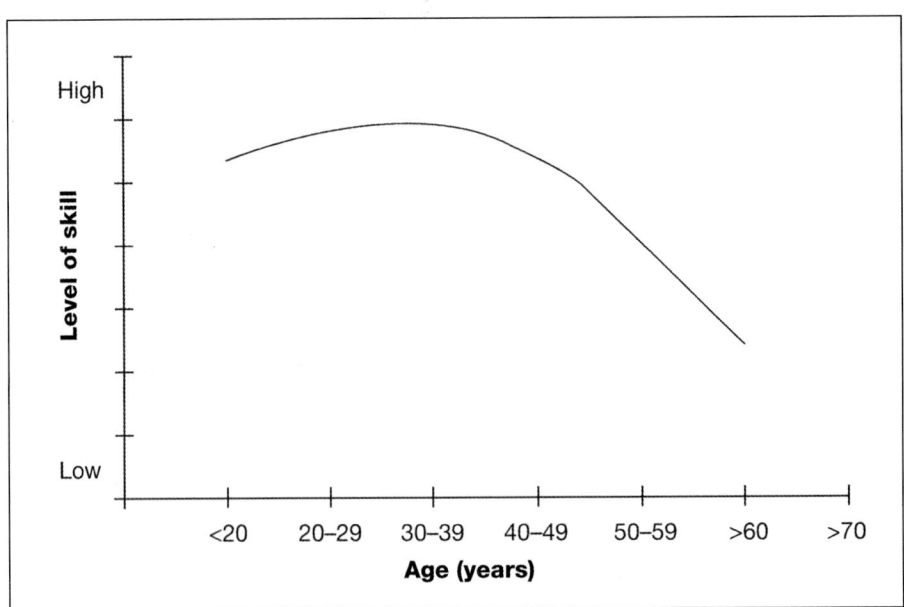

It is important to bear in mind that a high proportion of older adults with Down syndrome do not suffer from any significant physical and medical problems which can affect their self-care and independence skills. A few can survive into their 70s without any significant health issues. Bert Holbrook, aged 83 years, was identified as the world's oldest man with Down syndrome in November 2008.

With good health care support and the opportunities for lifelong learning and to live an active life in their local community people with Down syndrome can enjoy a good quality of life.

Chapter 2

Growth and nutrition

Growth and nutrition relate to the use of food for optimum physical and mental growth. A good diet requires a balance of proteins, carbohydrates, fats, vitamins, minerals, fibre and water. Such essentials are obtained from a wide variety of food types which includes milk and milk products, vegetables, fruits, bread, cereals, meat and eggs. For people with Down syndrome physical and mental growth has been shown to be delayed. Inadequate nutritional status may prove to be a significant factor causing this.

Stature

Growth charts for children and young adults with Down syndrome, from birth to eighteen years of age, are now widely available. Such charts are not available for adults over eighteen. Adults with Down syndrome are generally shorter compared to the general population. The life-span curve for the average age-related height for adults with Down syndrome is similar in shape to that for the general population but, as expected, is significantly lower at all ages (Figure 2). Men with Down syndrome are taller than women with Down syndrome of the same age, by on average, seven centimetres. The peak in height appears to occur around the late twenties to mid-thirties, some 5-10 years later than that for the general population. Similar to the general population, after middle-age, there is a slow reduction in height with increasing age. The height of an adult with Down syndrome must be compared to other adults with Down syndrome of the same sex and age and not with that of the general adult population, before unnecessary anxiety is raised regarding a person's short stature. Growth hormone therapy has been given to children with Down syndrome to improve their height. However, such therapy remains controversial and is of no proven benefit in adults (Chapter 14).

Figure 2 **Average height distribution for Down syndrome and general population**

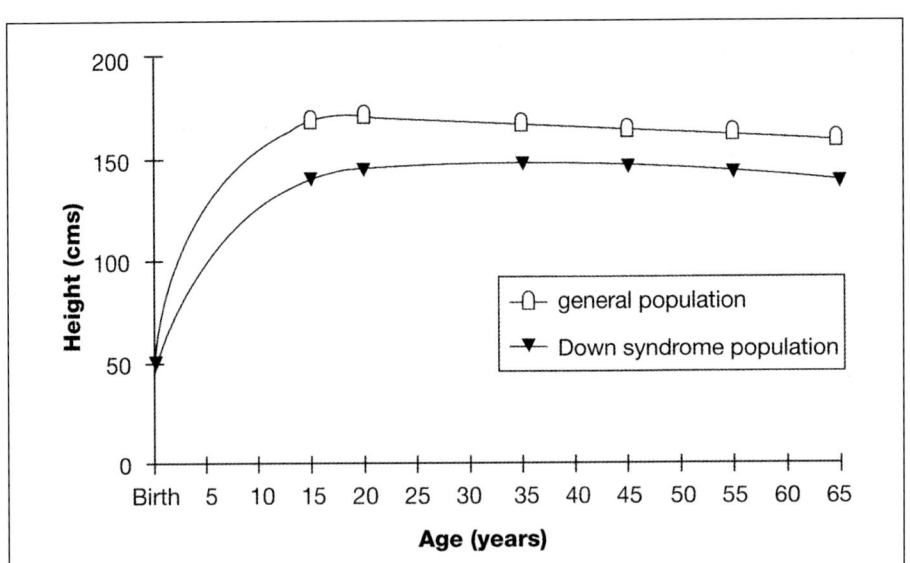

Obesity

Obesity is an increase in body weight beyond that which is necessary for one's height, as a result of excess body fat. It is a more severe form of being overweight. A standard way of measuring obesity is to use 'body mass index' (BMI) which is accepted to be a reasonable measure of the degree of body fat present. This is the weight in kilograms divided by the square of the height in metres (weight in kg/height in metres^2). The different levels of obesity are given in table 1.

Table 1 **Body Mass Index (BMI)***

Body Mass Index (BMI)*	
Underweight	less than 21
Desirable weight	21–24
Overweight	25–29
Obese	30–34
Medically significant obesity	35–39
Super-obesity	40–44
Morbid obesity	more than 44

*BMI=weight (kg)/height (m2)

Obesity is a common problem for the general population and this is also true for people with Down syndrome (Figure 3). In the general population 34% of adult males and 24% of adult females are said to be overweight (BMI 25-29). Six per cent of males and 8% of females are reported to be obese (BMI greater than 30). Among the Down syndrome adult population only 12% have 'desirable weight' (BMI 21-24), 29% have been shown to be 'overweight' (BMI 25-29) and a further 48% 'obese' (BMI greater than 30). Twenty-five percent have levels of obesity at or above the 'medically significant' level (BMI greater than 35). For adults with Down syndrome being overweight or obese is a major problem at all ages, but in particular for younger adults.

Why people become obese remains unclear, but there is an imbalance of excess energy intake to energy loss. Obese people do not necessarily eat more than required. Generally for people with Down syndrome a number of factors are important including excessive calorie intake, low metabolic rate, less physical activity (associated with decreased muscle tone and delayed development), side-effects of medication and hormonal abnormalities (eg hypothyroidism). Heredity factors, emotional problems and the cultural setting are other important factors. Low blood levels of growth hormone as a cause has been excluded, although problems with insulin metabolism remain a possibility. Obesity often begins in early childhood with adult obesity reflecting childhood obesity.

Figure 3 **Distribution of average body mass by age and sex**

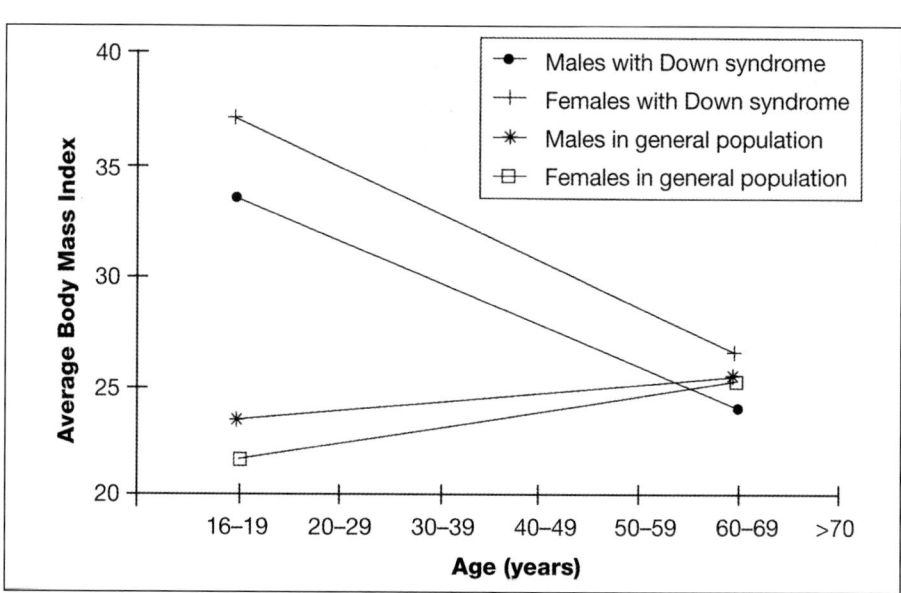

For any adult with Down syndrome who is suspected of being overweight or obese, their weight and if possible their calorie intake should be measured on a regular basis. An excessive increase in weight over a short period of time for no apparent reason should be investigated, eg for hypothyroidism. In common with the general population people with Down syndrome are susceptible to other complications associated with obesity. These include lung disease, arthritis (hands, knees, spine, and hips), diabetes, heart disease, hypertension, strokes, thyroid dysfunction, obstructive sleep apnoea, gallstones and digestive problems. It is important that people receive appropriate information, support and health care for these complications.

There are a number of popular magazines and books on dieting and how best to lose weight. The principles given generally apply also to adults with Down syndrome. These include the need for a change in diet, a change in behaviour with respect to food and support from others. It may be helpful for individuals to have the advice and support of a dietician. The only way to really lose weight is by a reduction in calorie intake and to increase exercise (especially aerobics which increases metabolic rate). Research studies in persons with Down syndrome show reduction in calorie intake and/or regular exercise over several weeks can significantly reduce obesity. Self-help groups and behavioural programmes recommended by health professionals can reinforce and help to maintain motivation. Drug therapies are available which can reduce appetite, but these are not recommended by doctors. Surgery, for example wiring of the jaws, removal of a part of the stomach to make the person feel 'full' quickly and reduction of the digestive system to reduce food absorption have been tried in the general population, but should not be performed on people with Down syndrome without expert medical advice. One problem is that dramatic weight loss will usually lead to weight being regained when normal dieting resumes. Better education and information for the person with Down syndrome, family members and paid staff to prevent obesity in the first place and improved access to health promotion can prevent future problems.

The importance of good nutrition

Good nutrition helps us to:

- maintain and improve our quality of life
- recover and heal after illness or an accident
- have a strong immune system to fight infection
- maintain our strength and energy
- reduce constipation, diarrhoea
- reduce anxiety
- prevent wasting of muscle
- maintain our weight and keep our mood stable

People with Down syndrome may have lower blood levels of some substances than the general population (for example calcium), have impaired glucose metabolism, altered uric acid and zinc levels or lower levels of some enzymes. It remains important to compare findings for any one person with Down syndrome to those for the Down syndrome population. A low measure may be normal for a person with Down syndrome. Wasted time and considerable distress can be caused by fruitless investigations looking for a reason when something is found to be apparently 'abnormal'. Medical advice from a specialist who cares for adults with Down syndrome should be sought if there are any concerns regarding nutritional deficiency or if abnormalities are found on routine tests. Certainly if there are other associated symptoms or signs then an expert opinion should be sought.

A deficiency of carbohydrates and/or proteins is unlikely to occur in Western countries. However it may occur where there is a restriction of diet, for example due to food fads or a loss of interest in food following a medical illness. The older anticonvulsant drugs (eg Phenytoin, Phenobarbitone) used to control epilepsy can lead to folate deficiency. If this is present, replacement therapy may be required. Maintaining a good diet should prevent nutritional deficiency.

Nutritional excess will occur if the calorie intake is greater than the amount of calories used up. This may lead to the development of obesity. Excessive intake of minerals and/or vitamins can lead to nutritional disorders, eg excessive salt intake can cause hypertension and excessive vitamin intake can cause nerve damage.

Vitamins and targeted nutritional intervention
(specially formulated combination of vitamins, minerals, hormones, enzymes, and amino acid supplements)

Megavitamin therapy to improve the intelligence, speech, height, health of children with Down syndrome has been previously advocated, but research has generally failed to confirm these claims. Some studies have reported benefit from vitamin supplementation on immune function with a possible greater resistance to infections. Other studies have found no improvement in mental ability or behaviour. The role of selenium (a mineral) and vitamin E (an antioxidant) in reducing effects of ageing are being investigated. At present, research does not support the use of such supplements. Although some clinicians have claimed an improvement in intelligence and in physical appearance, results from accepted research studies of targeted nutritional intervention are awaited. Nutritional and dietary supplements (eg Nutrivene-D) are now commercially marketed for persons with Down syndrome, but at present no nutritional substance can definitely be advocated to improve intelligence or general health in people with Down syndrome. A specialist medical opinion is advisable.

Healthy eating
Food is essential for survival as it gives the body the energy needed for growth and for leading an active life. Healthy eating enables people to access a better quality of life by reducing the risk of serious physical and psychological problems. There are also many social benefits of being fit and well and feeling good.

Overweight and obesity is probably the most obvious outcome of unhealthy eating. A balanced diet is the best means of keeping weight in proportion to one's height. We are all familiar with what foods are supposed to constitute a healthy diet and what foods we should avoid, or at least go carefully on.

The guidelines for a healthy diet are:

- eat a variety of foods
- eat plenty of foods rich in starch and fibre, such as wholemeal bread, potatoes, pasta, cereals
- eat fruit or vegetables each day
- maintain a diet containing a balance of vitamins and minerals
- don't eat too much fat or too many sugary things
- keep within the recommended limits for alcohol
- keep to appropriate portions
- take small steps to improve diet and weight rather than trying a 'quick fix'
- drink reasonable but not excessive amounts of water per day

Above all, enjoy your food!

Individuals with Down syndrome can learn good eating habits when their diet includes a variety of healthy foods at each mealtime. Variety can include: lean meats or meat substitutes, fruits and vegetables in a variety of colours, whole grain breads, cereals and pastas and milk or milk products such as yogurt and cheese. Involving individuals in meal planning has been shown to aid healthy eating. The importance of the 'family meal' must not be under-estimated as others can be models of good eating behaviour and it is often a good time to interact and 'catch-up'.

Keeping to a 'healthy weight' is sometimes difficult. If extra advice and help is required it is possible to contact a State Registered Dietician. Dieticians may be contacted through your GP's practice or by referral to an NHS Trust. Keeping to a sensible weight has many advantages and it's better to tackle the issue sooner rather than later. People with Down syndrome have a tendency to suffer from hypothyroidism which can lead to putting on extra weight, so regular health checks are essential.

There is lots of information and advice about healthy eating and dieting at www.nhs.uk/livewell

Chapter 3

Health professionals and support services

People with Down syndrome are entitled to the same standard of health care as everyone else. Unfortunately, not all health care professionals are knowledgeable about their general and particular health needs. In some situations health care professionals fail to make the reasonable adjustments needed to facilitate good health care for people with a learning disability. Sadly then the onus falls on the person's family members and/or paid staff, to obtain appropriate attention and care, especially if the person with Down syndrome has difficulty describing the source of pain or discomfort. In such cases it can be helpful to have a good knowledge of what various professionals can offer and where to go for help. Many family members and paid staff will have learned this from experience, but the information in this chapter may be of help to others.

As was explained in the introduction of this book, adults with Down syndrome are more likely than other people to suffer from a range of illnesses and medical conditions that require treatment. Particular physical disorders include sensory impairment, overweight and obesity, and thyroid dysfunction. Particular psychiatric disorders include dementia, depression and obsessive-compulsive disorders. This does not mean that all adults with Down syndrome will develop these disorders, but it does mean that health services should be aware of their diagnosis, treatment and management. Some people with Down syndrome find it difficult to communicate any pain or discomfort associated with a given illness. If ill-health is missed or misdiagnosed, much suffering may be caused which could have been avoided. For these reasons, people with Down syndrome should receive regular health checks as recommended by the Royal College of General Practitioners. You can find out more at www.rcgp.org.uk

Appendix B gives details about the important aspects of health which should be checked on a regular basis.

Resources which might be useful
Some people with Down syndrome may be worried about going to the doctors. Some may not understand what will happen and therefore may be uncooperative and anxious. This then causes anxiety for family members and paid staff and most importantly, lessens the likelihood that they will receive proper care and attention. Understanding and skill on the part of health care professionals can go a long way to reducing fears, but so can good preparation and support, for example asking for longer doctor's appointments or being seen first or last.

There are some useful Easy Read books available that explain to the person with Down syndrome what will happen. Some are suitable for children and some for adults. An example of the latter is *Going to the Doctor* published by Books Beyond Words. This book and others in the series can be used by family members and support staff, in collaboration with the person with a learning disability. It is also a useful resource for GPs and the primary care team. It emphasises the issue of consent and provides pictures that help to clarify the choices open to the patient. Many organisations for people with a learning disability have produced booklets that describe what happens when receiving treatments, by means of signs, symbols and drawings. Some booklets have been produced by people with a learning disability who understand the needs of others; there are more details in Appendices D and E.

If individuals, family carers or members of the public are concerned about treatment received in England they can find out about their rights and responsibilities from the NHS Constitution. For more information go to www.nhs.uk. People can also find out how to make a complaint about the organisation providing their treatment. Easy Read versions of all complaints procedures should be available. Similarly, for people in Scotland *The Charter of Patients' Rights and Responsibilities* from www.scotland.gov.uk explains to the public about their rights to health care and how to make comments, raise concerns or make a complaint. Information about complaints procedures in Northern Ireland can be found at http://bit.ly/1gP44yp.

The website http://www.wales.nhs.uk/sitesplus/899/home provides information about patients' rights and complaints procedures in Wales.

Health Professionals

The general practitioner (GP)

For the majority of people with Down syndrome, the main provider of health care is their general practitioner (GP), along with other professionals who together make up the primary health care team. GPs are easily accessible (or should be so). Usually the GP knows the family, may know the person with Down syndrome and may have always looked after them.

Many GP practices are supported by a team of other health care professionals (the primary health care team mentioned above) and it is becoming increasingly common to find that a range of services is offered at health centres. If this is the situation in your area, it can be very helpful to have the services of nurses, health visitors, physiotherapists, chiropodists, social workers and a pharmacy all under one roof. Travelling around in order to obtain different services can be costly, time consuming and tiring but, as yet, by no means everyone has access to a 'supermarket' type of primary health care. It is useful to know which professionals provide which service.

The NHS system in England went through a huge change in April 2013. Clinical commissioning groups, led by GPs have been given the responsibility of 'buying' services for their patients. More than ever, GPs now have a significant influence on which health services will be available to their patients in the future. The concern is that those with a lesser voice, eg persons with a learning disability, will lose their health services due to the 'free market'.

Paediatricians

Paediatricians are doctors who specialise principally in child health, but may also see young adults with Down syndrome. They assess, diagnose and care for children from young babies through to older teenagers with medical and developmental problems. Multi-professional community paediatric services are responsible for monitoring the development of children and young adults with learning difficulties. The paediatrician works in conjunction with health visitors, school nurses, speech and language therapists, occupational therapists and physiotherapists.

Paediatricians can arrange for the appropriate transfer of medical care of a young adult with Down syndrome from children's to adult health services.

Such transfers should be initiated and discussed at least one year before implementation. This gives time to coordinate with other support services such as education, social services and employment.

Psychiatrists

Psychiatrists in learning disability have particular expertise in the physical and mental health problems associated with learning disability. Since adults with Down syndrome are at greater risk than the general population of developing an emotional or psychological disorder (see Chapter 15) it is important to obtain specialist advice on diagnosis, cause, assessment, appropriate treatment and outlook. Some psychiatrists do undertake routine health screening, although this is more likely undertaken by GPs.

Community learning disability team (CLDT)

These teams have been set up to serve the particular needs of people with a learning disability and their family members, family carers and paid staff. Some teams are very small while others contain several professionals such as a psychiatrist, psychologist, occupational therapist, speech and language therapist, in addition to community nurses and social workers. Professionals in the team will understand the health care needs of people with a learning disability and can provide valuable support. Regular meetings are held by the team to discuss in a multi-professional forum the needs of each person with a learning disability in contact with the services.

Community learning disability nurses

Community nurses in learning disability teams (CLDTs) can give support and advice to adults with Down syndrome and their family members or to paid support staff. If necessary, a nurse from the community learning disability team can accompany the person with Down syndrome to the GP surgery to explain about particular health concerns. Community nurses can help with aspects such as supervision of medication, responding to mental health and epilepsy needs, knowledge of day services, obesity, continence and developing packages of care. Community nurses and other members of the team can put you in touch with other services, if required.

Social workers/care managers

Although social workers are not directly concerned with health care, attention to the social wellbeing of the person with Down syndrome and his or her family members or paid staff is essential for a satisfactory and satisfying life style.

If not based in the CLDT, social workers with expertise in learning disability may be based in social services teams in the community, sometimes in a local health centre or in a team attached to specialist services. They are responsible for assessing the needs of both the person with Down syndrome and of family carers. They can give information on local services to meet the person's needs, welfare benefits, housing options and assistive technology. Social workers or care managers can work with people with Down syndrome and their families if they have a personal budget to help them explore how best to spend their budget to meet their needs.

Physiotherapists
Many physiotherapists now work in GP surgeries or health centres and visit people's homes to provide advice and treatment. Using various techniques, such as exercise, electrotherapy and acupuncture they can help with a wide range of joint problems, chest conditions, continence care, pain or difficulties in movement and lack of balance and control of limbs.

Occupational therapists
The occupational therapist aims to assess the general level of function of each person in the areas of self-care, productivity or work activity and occupational skills – areas of importance to the general wellbeing, independence and development of a person with a learning disability. Occupational therapists usually work as part of a multidisciplinary CLDT or for an NHS trust and offer guidance and advice to individuals and families as well as for carrying out therapeutic programmes.

Speech and language therapists
Speech and language therapists are trained in the assessment of communication (verbal and non-verbal), in speech and language disorders and in the application of many varied treatments to enable a person with a learning disability to function as well as possible in his or her environment. Stammering, articulation difficulties, eating, drinking, swallowing and voice disorders are some of the issues that can be helped by speech and language therapy. Training and supervision of support workers in relation to communication issues is also an important role of the therapist.

Psychologists

Psychologists work as part of a team with professionals from other disciplines to promote the psychological wellbeing of people with a learning disability and to reduce psychological distress. They work with issues such as challenging behaviour, mental health needs such as anxiety and depression, and can provide grief and bereavement support as well as assessment and support for parenting, relationships and for people with dementia. They can also carry out holistic assessments of people's abilities and needs – for example whether they have a learning disability, an autistic spectrum condition etc.

Dieticians

A state registered dietician can assess the nutritional adequacy of a given diet and give detailed advice. Because of the dangers and disadvantages of obesity, which have been mentioned earlier, it is important that people with Down syndrome follow a healthy dietary regime that does not contribute to excess weight. The aim is to give people a consistent and practical message about healthy eating. The British Dietetic Association can provide names of both NHS and private dieticians working in your area.

Pharmacists

Pharmacists, also known as chemists, are health care professionals who practise in the field of the safe and effective use of medication. The role of the pharmacist has shifted from the traditional dispensing role to being an integrated member of the health care team directly involved in patient care. They can advise on 'over-the-counter' medication and can check that the medication prescribed by a doctor is appropriate and at the correct dosage. Many pharmacists now advise doctors on which is the most suitable and cost effective drug to prescribe.

Other services which offer support

A wide range of additional services are available for all adults, including adults with Down syndrome. These will vary from country to country, and from region to region. Although they may be provided in different settings they are available everywhere. They include:

Hearing aid or audiology services
The NHS audiology and hearing aid service is free and includes testing, the provision, fitting and servicing of hearing aids, and the provision of batteries. If in doubt about whether or not someone with Down syndrome is hearing well, the first place to go for assistance is the GP who will probably refer the person to a hearing aid centre or to a hospital ear, nose and throat (ENT) department. Professionals at audiology and hearing aid centres may need support to meet the needs of a person with a learning disability. In this case it can be useful to contact an audiologist or hearing therapist with experience in this field. They can provide valuable help with assessment and supporting the person to get full benefit from their hearing aid. Other people, such as nurses working in CLDTs or specialist social workers, may also have experience in helping people to get maximum benefit from a hearing aid. They may also be able to advise about assistive technology and communication support. Action on Hearing Loss formerly the Royal National Institute for the Deaf can also provide extra advice and support.

Services for people who are visually impaired
Some visual impairments are very common amongst people with Down syndrome and it is important that advice should be sought promptly if a visual impairment is suspected. Routine visits to the optometrist (person trained to examine and test eyes and prescribe correcting lenses) should be made to check on visual acuity (sharpness of vision), on the correct deviation of light by the lens of the eye, on cataracts and other eye conditions.

As with hearing problems, help and advice is available from your GP and members of the community learning disability team. A home visit from an optometrist can be arranged if necessary. Apart from glasses, low vision aids, including hand and stand magnifiers can be prescribed through the NHS.

Professional help and training may be needed to help some people with Down syndrome to make the most of restricted vision. The Royal National Institute of Blind People (RNIB) and the Partially Sighted Society provides information on mobility aids, benefits, technology, social services and education.

Dental care services

Many people are able to receive dental treatment from their local dentist as long as adjustments are made to meet the person's needs. Some people with Down syndrome may need to have treatment from a community dentist with additional training who is able to meet their particular needs, However many family members and paid staff report difficulty in finding one locally. Many areas have at least one senior dentist with experience of providing dental care for people with a learning disability, but this service is not always well publicised.

Short break services

These offer an opportunity for adults with Down syndrome to spend time away from their families. This enables the family to 'have a break' and the person with Down syndrome to have time with others outside the family and possibly become more independent. Short breaks are usually paid for by health or social services and provided by the local authority or by private or voluntary sector organisations. Short break services vary from local authority to local authority. You can find out more from your local authority, care manager, social worker or from other professionals who are providing support.

Day centres

Day centres were in the past places where people with a learning disability could go to meet each other and take part in different activities. Many large day centres are now being closed and there is a much more diverse and person centred range of support available to people with a learning disability. Many smaller centres still offer a choice of activities, eg arts and crafts, sports, computers, health and beauty, games. Individual budgets have opened up greater opportunities in ordinary community settings. Many more people with learning disabilities now work in paid or voluntary jobs, attend college or adult education classes and have greater access to community leisure facilities.

Down syndrome organisations

These have usually been formed by parents of children with Down syndrome and are able to provide a wide range of support through newsletters, meetings, literature and funding of research (see Appendix E for details).

Other voluntary organisations
There are many organisations which can provide help for people with a disability. Appendix E lists the contact details of many such organisations. If the one you are looking for is not listed, it may be helpful to try your local public library. Local centres for independent living or a local council for disabled people in your area may be able to provide advice on a wide range of services and support including details about managing a personal budget, providers, clubs and activities The internet

The internet
The internet can be a good source of information for people with Down syndrome, family members and support staff; however it is essential that you are able to determine which sources are credible. When looking for information on the internet you need to critically weigh up its worth as not everything is up to date or based on good evidence.

Some organisations have excellent sites with information as well as opportunities for people to share their stories, ask questions and share ideas.

When assessing information from the internet think about who has produced the information, when it was written, if it is current or obsolete, objective and reliable. Some websites are listed in appendix E.

Specific medical issues

The next section of the book gives information about various treatments which may be used to treat specific medical conditions. There is a brief description of the condition, possible causes, symptoms, the range of possible treatments and any complications which may, on occasion, result from the condition. It also highlights which conditions are more likely to be experienced by people with Down Syndrome or which are likely to be more serious in people with Down Syndrome. It isn't, of course, a substitute for medical referral and treatment, but can help alert people with Down syndrome, family members or paid staff to particular conditions. If there are ongoing concerns, the person and those who support them are advised to consult their GP.

Chapter 4

Vision and related issues

The shape of the eyes is often the first indication that a new-born baby may have Down syndrome. In adults with Down syndrome abnormalities of the eye (Figure 4) can occur, with the commonest due to errors of focussing including short-sightedness and long-sightedness. Some features of the eyes cause no significant problems (eg upward slanting eyes or speckling of the iris) whilst others can impair vision significantly, for example cataracts and glaucoma. Many eye problems increase with age and may remain undetected for some time leading to particular physical, mental, educational and social difficulties. Good vision is important for enabling someone to maintain independence and general wellbeing.

Minor impairments in vision in an individual with Down syndrome can significantly affect their quality of life. Family members and paid support staff must be aware that eye problems are more common in adults with Down syndrome, mainly due to premature ageing. It is important, therefore, for regular screening for visual and related problems to be undertaken. The earlier a problem is identified the better the outlook after treatment. **If there is any concern a doctor's opinion should always be sought.** An assessment by an ophthalmologist or eye specialist may be required and should include testing for visual acuity (ability to see clearly) and for glaucoma (see below), examination of the retina (back of the eye) and of the lens of the eye for cataracts (see below).

Figure 4 **The different parts of an eye**

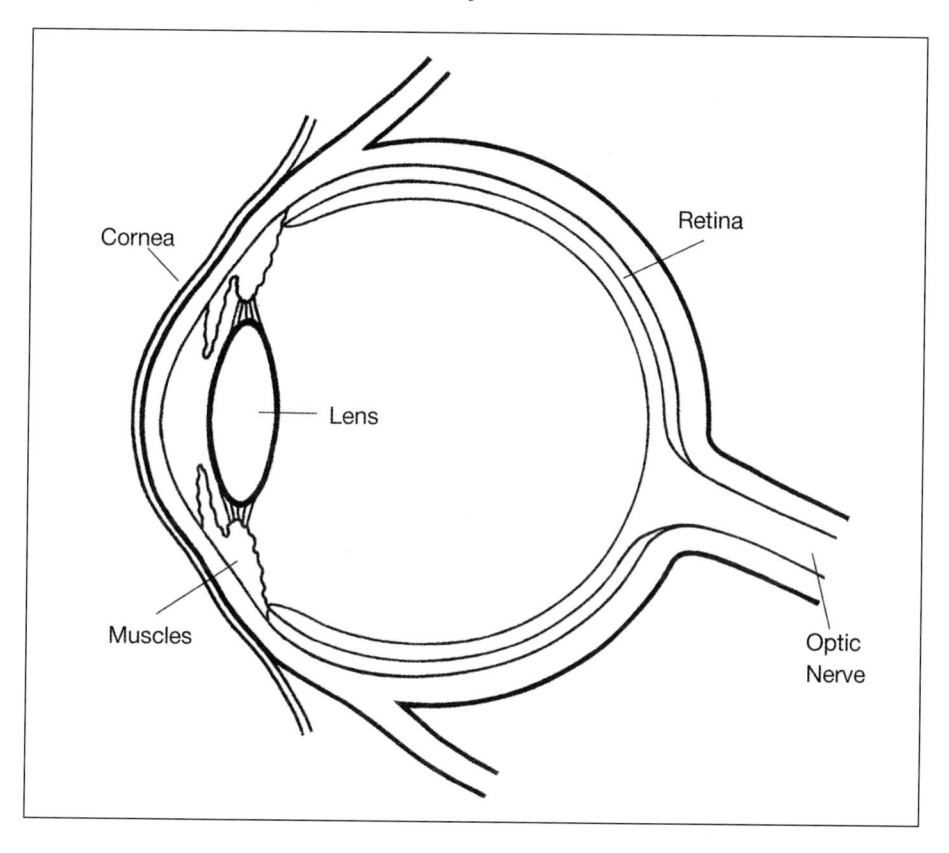

[Diagram of an eye labeled with: Cornea, Lens, Muscles, Retina, Optic Nerve]

Short-sightedness (myopia)

Causes: The focusing power of the eyes is too strong leading to light rays being brought to a focus in front of the retina (back of the eye) rather than on the retina, as should happen.

Symptoms and signs: The person has difficulty in seeing, but this is often not reported by individuals or detected by family members or paid staff. Close objects are still seen clearly, but objects further away are blurred and not in focus. Symptoms can include eyestrain, headaches, changes in day-to-day activities or changes in behaviour. There might also be emotional changes.

Investigations: The assessment of vision by an optometrist (person trained to examine and test eyes and prescribe correcting lenses) or by the hospital eye department is required if loss in vision is suspected. Time and patience is required for a successful assessment.

Complications: There are usually no complications, but occasionally short sightedness can lead to an increase in accidents such as trips and falls or misdiagnosis of changes in behaviour, eg those caused by a mental health problem such as depression or dementia.

Treatment and prevention: The prescribing of glasses or contact lenses is now standard. Fitting and getting the person to wear them can, however, be difficult due to the individual finding them uncomfortable or the brain being unable to adjust to the improvement in vision. Breakage or loss can be a problem and it is recommended that a spare set is readily available.

Surgery is increasingly used as an effective alternative to wearing glasses or lenses. LASIK (laser assisted in-situ keratomileusis), PRK (photorefractive keratectomy) and LASEK (laser assisted sub-epithelial keratectomy) aim to change the focusing power of the cornea. The use of visual aids and modification to the environment (eg greater use of lighting and colour) and regular outdoor physical activity can be of considerable benefit. Regular check-ups (every 1-2 years) are recommended.

Long-sightedness (hypermetropia)
Causes: The focusing power of the eyes is too weak. Light rays are brought to a focus behind the retina and not on it.

Symptoms and signs: As with short-sightedness, problems may not be reported by individuals or detected by family carers and paid staff. Usually there is difficulty in seeing close objects in focus although far vision can also be affected. Occasionally eyestrain and headaches can occur. A squint can develop and the eyes appear to look in different directions.

Investigations: See short-sightedness (above).

Complications: Usually none but there is an increased risk of glaucoma developing.

Treatment and prevention: See short-sightedness (above).

Astigmatism
A condition of the eye where the surface of the cornea is not smoothly 'spherical'.

Causes: Often the cause is unknown. The condition can be present at birth or can occur because of other eye problems eg keratoconus (below).

Symptoms and signs: Difficulty in seeing may not be reported by individuals or detected by family members or paid support staff. It can include blurring of vision, eyestrain and headaches.

Investigations/ Complications/Treatment: See short-sightedness (above). A particular form of glasses is required.

Accommodation (Abnormal)

The inability of the eye to change focus correctly in order that both near and far objects can be seen clearly and in focus.

Causes: This condition is due to the impairment in the elasticity of the eye lens and impairment in the action of the muscles of the eye. It can be present in newborn babies with Down syndrome.

Symptoms and signs: The person usually has difficulty in focusing on close objects.

Investigations/Complications/Treatment: See short-sightedness (above).

Squint (Strabismus)

The deviation of one eye from the other eye, pointing inwards (esotropia), pointing outwards (exotropia), upwards (hypertropia) and downwards (hypotropia). This is extremely common in people with Down syndrome. A squint can lead to the brain receiving two images and ignoring images from one eye ('lazy eye').

Causes: The condition is thought to be due to an imbalance of the eye muscles, it is often present at birth and is seldom due to an underlying eye or brain disorder.

Symptoms and signs: Usually the eye(s) turn in. Occasionally the eye(s) turn out. Depth perception can be impaired leading to problems with walking up or down stairs and with fine motor skills. The squint may be constant or intermittent and generally worsens when a person is tired.

Investigations: A squint is detected by 'corneal reflection' where reflection from a bright light falls symmetrically on each cornea if the person has no squint and asymmetrically if a squint is present. Further investigations are usually not required unless a squint occurs when previously one was not present. Investigation may be needed to establish whether there is any underlying problem, eg nerve palsy. A squint should be detected as part of a health screening assessment.

Complications: A squint can lead to deterioration in vision in the 'lazy eye'.

Treatment: Usually no treatment is given in adulthood. In childhood the refractive state of the eye requires assessment and glasses are worn to correct any error. Wearing an eye patch on the good eye allows muscles in the bad eye to strengthen. Where possible surgery or botulinim toxin injections can be carried out.

Inflammation of the eyelids (blepharitis)

Causes: A common condition, which is usually due to a bacterial infection or skin conditions. The risk of an infection is increased if there is a blockage of the duct draining tears, dry eyes or a skin disease in an adult with Down syndrome.

Symptoms and signs: Usually there is a red eyelid margin, irritable eyelids, a burning sensation in the eye and dry flakes on the eyelid.

Investigations: Usually none are required as the diagnosis can be made just by observation.

Complications: Rubbing of the eyes can lead to the eyelid turning out or turning in. Ingrowing eyelashes can occur or, in a few cases, conjunctivitis (below) can also develop. Repeated episodes are not uncommon and bacterial infections can be spread to other people.

Treatment and prevention: The eyelids need to be kept clean and the person with the eye infection needs to be encouraged to not rub or touch their eyes. Any crusts present should be removed with warm water or cotton wool swabs dipped in a dilute solution of sodium bicarbonate or in baby shampoo. Antibiotic ointment or weak steroids can be used. Any underlying skin, dry eyes or scalp problem that is present will also require treatment.

Conjunctivitis
An inflammation of the membrane covering the eye.

Causes: Conjunctivitis is usually due to a bacterial or viral infection. Other causes can include an allergy (increased sensitivity to a substance), something in the eye and excessive wearing of contact lenses.

Symptoms and signs: The commonest symptom is bilateral red eyes. Other symptoms include a weeping eye, an uncomfortable feeling in the eye, a sticky eye, itching and blurring of vision.

Investigations: None required.

Complications: There may be recurrent infections.

Treatment and prevention: The person needs to avoid rubbing the eye as this will lead to the infection spreading. Treatment is with topical antibiotics (eg Chloramphenicol eye drops). If the conjunctivitis is due to an allergy, antihistamine drops or sodium cromoglycate may help. If symptoms continue, the person may need a referral to an ophthalmologist. If it is due to a foreign body, remove the offending particle if possible or seek medical help if necessary. If it recurs and the person wears contact lenses then it may be necessary to change the type of contact lenses being worn.

Cataracts

An opacity of the clear focussing lens of the eye. Cataracts can be in one or both eyes.

Causes: The condition can be present at birth. There is a greater risk with increasing age due to changes in the protein in the lens of the eye. Occasionally a cataract can be due to the presence of glaucoma (below) or diabetes (Chapter 14).

Symptoms and signs: The person will experience gradual loss of vision, 'cloudy' lens, though, not associated with pain in the eye. See short-sightedness (above).

Investigations: The presence of a grey/white pupil can be seen on examination. The assessment of any underlying impaired vision by an optometrist (person trained to examine and test eyes and prescribe correcting lenses) or by the hospital eye department is required.

Complications: See short-sightedness (above).

Treatment: Good lighting and spectacles may be of benefit when the condition is not too severe. For severe cases or when symptoms restrict lifestyle, surgery should be offered. Surgery on a cataract is usually a day case procedure under local anaesthetic. The lens can be removed and an artificial lens implanted. Full activities can usually be resumed the next day. If the surgery is more complicated antibiotics and anti-inflammatory eye drops need to be applied post operatively. Vision is usually greatly improved, however not entirely normal and the person may still require glasses for near vision.

Glaucoma
An increase in the pressure within the eye leading to impaired vision. Can be sudden or gradual.

Causes: Often no cause can be found. It can be associated with long-sightedness (above), diabetes (Chapter 14) or trauma to the eye.

Symptoms and signs: When gradual in onset, usually no difficulty is experienced and the condition is picked up at routine screening. Symptoms can include increased production of tears, rubbing of eyes, swelling of cornea, closure of the eye, inability to tolerate light, impaired vision and pain in the eye.

Investigations: An ophthalmologist or an eye specialist assessment is required. The pressure within the eye needs to be measured and the eyes examined for further damage.

Complications: Optic nerve damage with loss of vision can occur.

Treatment: The pressure within the eye needs to be reduced. This can be done by using medication (eye drops), laser treatment or by surgery. If it presents acutely admission to hospital and intravenous medications may be required.

Keratoconus
Conical protrusion of the central part of the cornea due to thinning of the cornea. It can affect both eyes at the same time and usually gets worse over time.

Causes: Often the cause is unknown, but the condition can occur due to excessive rubbing of the eyes.

Symptoms and signs: See short-sightedness (above). Protrusion may be seen from the side.

Investigations: The severity and the effect on vision should be assessed by an ophthalmologist.

Complications: If severe and untreated permanently impaired vision can occur.

Treatment: For an acute condition the person needs to treat their eye with eye lubricants, padding of the eye and pain relief. A chronic condition of keratoconus can be treated with glasses, hard contact lenses or by surgical intervention. If scarring is present a corneal transplant may be necessary. The person needs to be assessed for an underlying cause that may lead to excessive eye rubbing (eg dry eyes, allergies, cataracts, boredom, self-stimulation).

Nystagmus
Repetitive side to side movement usually of both eyes.

Causes: Usually the condition is present since birth but it can also be due to the side-effects of drugs.

Symptoms and signs: The commonest form is the constant horizontal vibrations of the eyes. Nystagmus is usually not painful.

Investigations: Usually no investigation is required unless the condition is due to an underlying cause or occurs when previously not present. It should be identified as part of the health screening assessment.

Complications: The vision can be affected. Unusual head postures can develop to reduce the effect of nystagmus.

Treatment: There is no need for medical intervention unless there is an underlying cause which requires treatment.

Retinal detachment
The retina becomes separated from other structures of the eye.

Causes: Often no cause is found. There is increased risk in people with short-sightedness, and post cataract surgery and in people who self-harm or show aggressive behaviour (eg head banging).

Symptoms and signs: See short-sightedness (above). There is sudden loss of a part of the visual field, or worsening vision. The person may experience flashes, spots, shapes or 'floaters' in front of their eye. It is often described as a curtain falling over the person's vision and is usually painless.

Investigations: Severity and the effect on vision should be assessed by an ophthalmologist.

Complications: Permanent loss of vision.

Treatment: If only a small area is affected close monitoring may be sufficient. In the case of a severe detachment then surgery, laser treatment or silicone implants will be necessary to reattach the retina.

Macular degeneration

Deterioration in the centre of the retina (macula).

Causes: The condition can be caused by premature ageing, and the increased growth of blood vessels into the macula.

Symptoms and signs: These include a blind spot in the central vision, dark, blurry areas or blind spots appearing in the centre of the person's vision, difficulty recognising people's faces, reading text or seeing the television clearly and a decline in day-to-day skills.

Investigations: Severity and the effect on vision should be assessed by an ophthalmologist.

Complications: Gradual loss of vision.

Treatment: Macular degeneration is not fully reversible. Using a laser (laser photocoagulation) to reduce the number of blood vessels around the macula can slow down the rate of progress of the disease. People usually compensate with large-print publications and magnifying lenses for everyday activities.
In addition, evidence suggests that certain vitamins and antioxidants - vitamins A, C and E, beta-carotene and zinc – may help to reduce the risk of severe vision loss. Research continues into the benefits of this therapy. Anti-vascular endothelial growth factor medication can be injected into the eye and used to slow down or prevent the growth of the abnormal blood vessels within the eye.

Chapter 5

Hearing and related issues

Hearing and ear related problems are often life-long issues for individuals with Down syndrome. Several difficulties are related to the structure of the ear in people with Down syndrome. The ear has three parts: outer, middle and inner (Figure 5). Sound enters the outer ear and moves through the ear canal to vibrate the eardrum and small bones in the middle ear. Vibrations are then passed on to the inner ear (cochlea) and are transmitted by a nerve (auditory nerve) to the hearing centre in the brain. Problems can occur anywhere along this pathway. As with visual problems, hearing problems may be difficult to detect and regular screening for hearing problems is therefore important. The earlier the identification of a problem the better the outlook after treatment. **If the person with Down syndrome, their family members or paid staff are concerned about a hearing problem then a doctor's opinion should always be sought.** An ear specialist's assessment may be required.

Figure 5 **Parts of the ear**

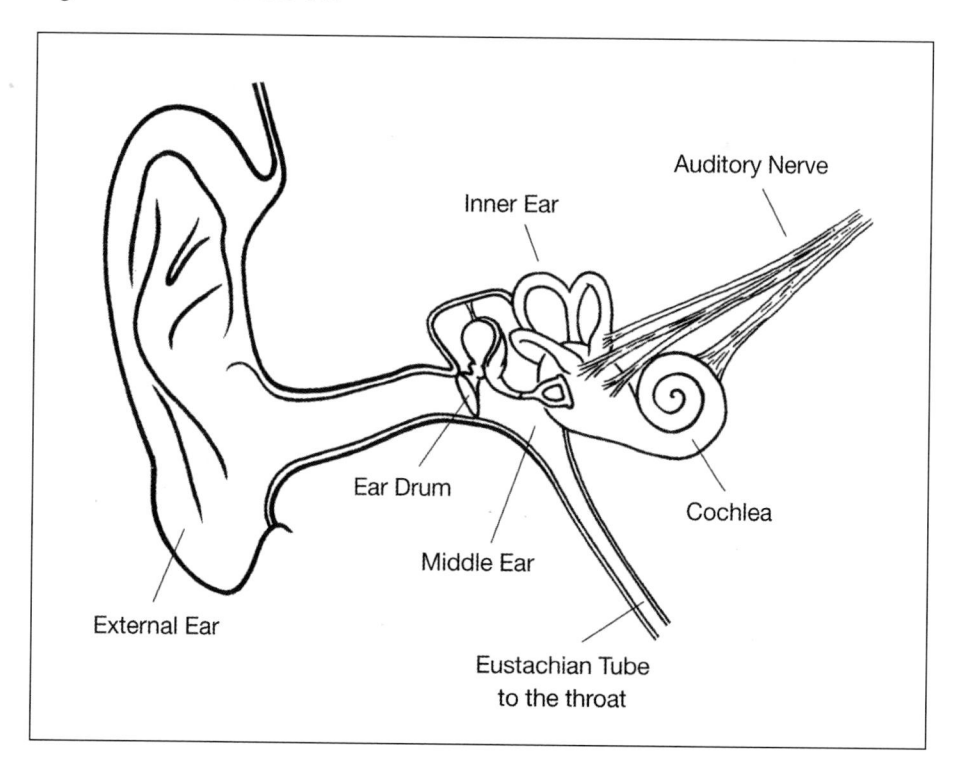

Hearing loss
Hearing loss will affect virtually all people with Down syndrome at some point in their lives. *Any* degree of hearing loss can be described as deafness.

There are two common forms of hearing loss: **conductive hearing loss** (where sound does not reach the inner ear appropriately) and **sensorineural hearing loss** (problems with the cochlea or with the auditory nerve carrying impulses to the brain area). A person can have both types at the same time. Temporary and permanent hearing loss can occur.

Causes: The commonest causes are impacted wax in the ear canal, 'glue ear' (below), and changes in the structures of the ear with age (presbycusis). Other important causes include recurrent middle ear infections (below), a perforated eardrum with damage to the middle ear, an object in the ear canal, a side effect of certain medications and rarely, disease affecting the auditory nerve.

Symptoms and signs: Often mild to moderate hearing loss can go unrecognised. With age, high pitched sounds are usually the first to be lost (eg 's' sounds). Hearing loss may be suspected if there is failure to respond to sound, problems in learning, being withdrawn, being quiet, not responding to communication and an increase in behavioural or emotional problems. A misdiagnosis of dementia can be made. Family members or paid staff may say 'he has selective hearing'.

Investigations: There will need to be an assessment for hearing loss after any wax present in the ear canal is removed. Hearing tests should be, where possible, carried out by an audiologist (a person who assesses hearing) with experience in seeing people with a learning disability. Good assessment of people with Down syndrome can require clear explanation to ensure cooperation and because people may have small ear canals, and/or excessive wax. Occasionally mild sedation may be required. **Any sudden unexplained hearing loss requires immediate referral.**

Complications: Problems that can occur include: impaired speech and language, poor educational progress, impaired social interaction, behavioural and emotional problems. A misdiagnosis of a mental health disorder (eg depression or dementia) can occur.

Treatment and prevention: Early detection is essential to prevent serious impairment and disability. Conductive deafness can often be improved. Provision of a hearing aid from a specialist centre (Chapter 3) is often necessary (see hearing aids below). It can be difficult for the person to accept wearing a hearing aid and considerable time and effort may be needed to encourage the person to wear an aid. If appropriate, recurrent upper respiratory tract infections, which lead to conductive hearing loss, may be treated with decongestants, large doses of vitamin C and antibiotics. Surgery may be used when there is a perforation of the ear drum.

Sensorineural deafness is usually permanent and is more difficult to manage. Some people can benefit from a cochlear implant, although following this, sounds heard are still not normal and the person will require training to interpret the new sounds. There are however other ways to improve understanding and communication. These are mainly by improving face-to-face communication, involving a speech and language therapist and/or by learning communication signs and symbols. Speaking in a quieter environment, speaking slowly and louder with the use of gestures or pictures are simple practical measures. Support for family members and paid staff is important in order to help the person understand and manage their deafness.

Earache
Pain in or around the ear.

Causes: This is usually caused by an inflammation or ear infection (below) of the outer or middle ear. Other causes can include 'glue ear' (below) and referred pain from the teeth, tonsils or sinuses.

Symptoms and signs: Earache can present as pain in the ear, discharge from the ear, the person pulling or rubbing their ear or banging their head on furniture. Other more general features are being distressed, disturbed sleep, refusing to eat, showing emotional or behaviour changes.

Investigations: There needs to be a careful medical examination of the ear and also the nose and throat.

Complications: Usually there are none. But if an infection is present, this can spread and can lead to conductive deafness (see hearing loss above).

Treatment: The cause needs to be found and treated. Painkillers (eg paracetamol) can relieve any discomfort. Any infection needs prompt treatment with antibiotics.

Impacted earwax (cerumen)

This is due to the build up of a yellow-brown secretion produced by glands in the outer ear. This is a normal product which usually helps to keep the ear canal clean.

Causes: The excessive production of ear wax is common in people with Down syndrome. The build up of wax is possibly due to the presence of smaller ear canals in people with Down syndrome. The risk of impaction increases with age.

Symptoms and signs: These include hearing loss (above), a feeling of being 'bunged up' and irritation in the ear.

Investigations: An ear examination will reveal impacted wax.

Complications: Impacted wax can result in a conductive hearing loss (above).

Treatment: Hard wax should be removed by a professional person after softening the wax with oil over several days and then flushing out with warm water (syringing of ears). Occasionally a probe may be needed to remove wax. The insertion of objects, such as ear buds, by the person or family members or paid staff can lead to wax being trapped further down the ear canal or can lead to a perforation of the ear drum.

Ear infections

Causes: An acute infection can either be viral or bacterial. A chronic ear infection often presents as a perforated ear drum with discharge from the middle ear. A middle ear infection is known as otitis media. External ear infections are called otitis externa.

Symptoms and signs: An acute infection presents with earache (above), discharge from ear, hearing loss (above), inflamed ear, fever and usually a history of a recent cold or of flu. Build up of fluid behind the eardrum can occur (serous otitis). A chronic condition usually has no redness or bulging of the eardrum and no pain, but the presence of 'glue ear' (below). Emotional or behavioural changes can be the first sign of an ear infection.

Investigations: An ear, nose and throat examination is necessary. A hearing assessment may be necessary if hearing loss persists.

Complications: Recurrent infections can lead to a 'glue ear' (below) or hearing loss (above).

Treatment: The underlying cause must be treated. Paracetamol can be given for pain. Antibiotics and decongestant drugs may be prescribed although many ear infections can get better without any intervention. Hearing will need to be monitored. In otitis externa it is important to keep the ear canal clean and antibiotic drops can be used.

Glue ear

A build up of thick and sticky fluid ('glue') in the middle ear. Common, especially in children.

Causes: Caused by a blockage of the Eustachian tube from the middle ear to the throat because of congestion during upper respiratory tract infections, which leads to a build up of 'glue-like' fluid in the middle ear.

Symptoms and signs: (See hearing loss above). Often there is no pain and therefore the condition goes undiagnosed.

Investigations: An ear, nose and throat examination and a hearing assessment will be required.

Complications: Glue ear can result in persistent hearing loss (above).

Treatment and prevention: In mild cases reassurance with review maybe enough as most cases tend to resolve after a few months. Decongestant medication taken for several weeks may be of benefit but may have limited effect. Surgical intervention can be given with the use of grommets and T tubes (tiny plastic washers inserted into the ear drum) to let air into the ear. This prevents the accumulation and development of the fluid. Insertion of tubes remains controversial and specialist advice should be sought. Follow up after insertion is required to monitor improvement. Grommets and tubes are designed to extrude as part of the natural cleaning process of the ear and review is necessary to assess the state of the middle ear when the tubes fall out. Hearing aids or removal of adenoids and/or tonsils may also be considered. Ear plugs should be worn at times of bathing and swimming to prevent water entering the middle ear through the tube.

Hearing aids

Hearing aids are used to amplify sound to the middle ear. They are usually worn behind the ear or in the ear. The hearing aid will help the person make better use of the hearing they have left. However, the quality of the sound the person hears through their hearing aid will not be the same as natural sound. Many people take some time to adapt to using a hearing aid and not all people will get used to it, including some people with Down syndrome. Advice from an audiologist or hearing therapist is often needed before and after fitting to support the person to adapt to the hearing aid (see Hearing aid services – Chapter 3). Ongoing training and support from a speech and language therapist may be necessary. In order to assess and encourage good communication, gradual introduction of the aid is usually recommended, initially in conversation with one person or listening to a favourite TV programme or music. A hearing therapist can advise family members and paid support staff about ways to adapt their verbal and non-verbal communication in order to support good communication with a person with a hearing loss.

As well as changing how people communicate with the person and exploring the use of a hearing aid, there are also many other products that can help improve the quality of life of a person with a hearing loss. These include, amplified phones, TV listeners, vibrating alarm clocks and flashing or vibrating door bells. More information can be obtained from the local hearing aid centre, from the person's audiologist or hearing therapist or from Action on Hearing Loss at www.actiononhearingloss.org.uk

Chapter 6

Heart and circulation

Heart and circulatory problems are very common in people with Down syndrome, approximately half of children with Down syndrome are born with a heart defect. Nowadays such problems are usually detected before or soon after birth. Problems can however persist into adulthood or start later in life and give cause for concern. Such problems can arise because of changes to the structure of the heart or are to do with the regular beating of the heart. As for children, all adults with Down syndrome should continue to have ongoing monitoring of the health of their heart. Regular screening for heart and circulation problems at all ages should be undertaken to detect any evidence that the heart is declining in its function. **If any symptoms or signs suggesting a heart problem are observed a medical opinion must be sought.**

Heart rate

The heart rate is detected by pressing one or more fingers against the skin over an artery (usually at the wrist, neck or groin). The rate can be measured as beats per minute and corresponds to the heart rate. The heart rate is usually between 60 and 100 beats per minute when a person is resting. For an adult in the general population the average heart rate is 72 beats per minute, but for adults with Down syndrome it is lower at 65 beats per minute. An abnormal heart rate (fast or slow); abnormal rhythm or a weak pulse can be a sign of heart disease, obstruction of the blood circulation or of general ill-health.

Causes: The heart rate can be higher (tachycardia, over 85 beats per minute) due to exercise, emotion, fever, anaemia, hyperthyroidism and heart disease. It can be lower (bradycardia, less than 50 beats per minute) due to hypothermia, hypothyroidism, drug therapy or heart disease.

Symptoms and signs: As well as a slow or fast heart rate there can be a number of other symptoms present. These include palpitations (a fluttering feeling in the chest), chest pain, fainting, breathlessness and poor exercise tolerance.

Investigations: These include examination of the health of the heart by electrocardiography (ECG, recording of the electrical currents of the heart) and echocardiography (ultrasound of the heart to produce moving images). Blood tests can also be undertaken to exclude illnesses that can affect the heart (eg thyroid disease, anaemia).

Complications: Problems may not occur, but heart failure and hypotension (low blood pressure) are important complications to watch out for.

Treatment: Any treatment given will depend on the underlying cause and also if there are secondary problems. Usually reassurance and an explanation of what is happening is all that is needed. However, medication to slow or increase the heart rate or to reduce the work on the heart is usually the main form of treatment, if intervention is required. Only rarely may a heart pacemaker need to be fitted if there is no improvement with medication or if the heart problem is life threatening.

Blood pressure

Blood pressure (BP) is the pressure exerted by the flow of blood through the arteries of the body. Pressure can vary considerably during different stresses put on the heart. The highest pressure point (systolic BP) is pressure created by the contraction of the heart muscle and the lowest point (diastolic BP) is that present when the heart muscle is in relaxation. No single BP is normal for all individuals in all circumstances. The average BP for a resting adult in the general population is a systolic BP of 110-120mmHg and a diastolic BP of 75-80mmHg. For an adult with Down syndrome it is a systolic BP of 105-115mmHg and a diastolic BP of 70-75mmHg respectively. For children and young adults the BP is lower. There is a gradual increase in BP with age (Figure 6). A normal BP can vary for many reasons including age, anxiety, exercise and with the size of the cuff used.

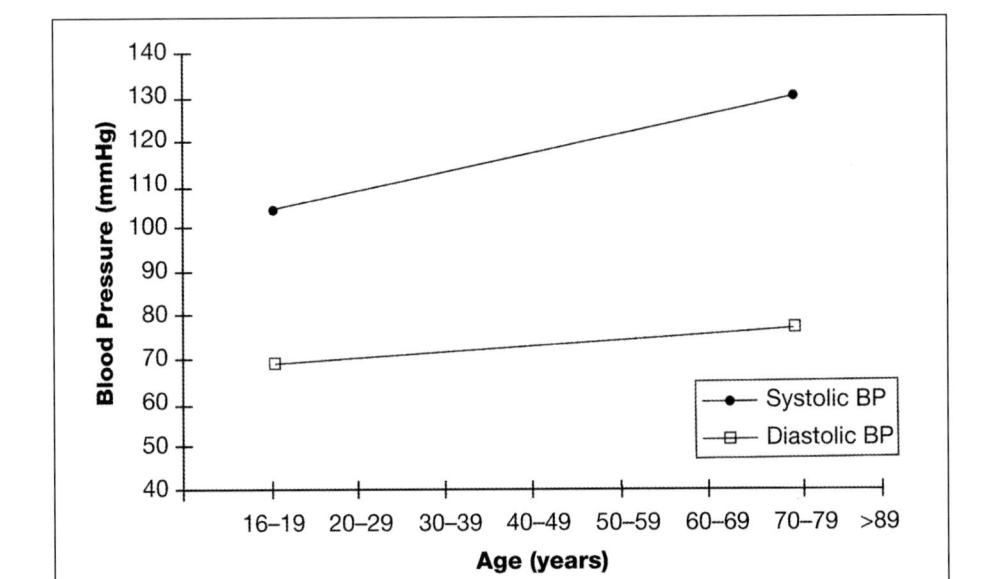

Figure 6 **Blood pressure by age for population of people with Down syndrome**

Hypertension (high blood pressure)

This is an uncommon condition in adults with Down syndrome. The BP must be measured on several occasions before it can be declared abnormally elevated (hypertensive). Hypertension for adults with Down syndrome is a systolic BP greater than 90mmHg plus age in years and/or a diastolic BP greater than 90mmHg.

Causes: In the vast majority of people no cause is found, but in a significant minority obesity, heart disease, kidney disease (eg narrowing of renal arteries), gland disorders (eg hyperthyroidism, Cushing's disease) and drugs (eg steroids) can be factors.

Symptoms and signs: Often there are no symptoms, but severe hypertension can present with headaches, shortness of breath, dizziness or confusion.

Investigations: Initially there is a need to measure the BP on several occasions to confirm a persistently high level. A general physical examination particularly including the heart, eyes, and urine is necessary to exclude any organ damage. Blood tests will be necessary to investigate for a possible underlying cause and to exclude kidney damage.

Complications: Not inevitable, but if uncontrolled for some time can lead to coronary heart disease, peripheral vascular disease, kidney failure, a stroke or impaired vision.

Treatment and prevention: Regular BP checks for all adults with Down syndrome, but in particular for those with a previous high level, should be undertaken. This can be done by the person's GP. A reduction in weight, reduced salt intake, exercise, relaxation and stopping smoking have been shown to be beneficial. Antihypertensive drugs (eg diuretics, beta-blockers) may be necessary. Any drug treatment will need to be monitored closely by a doctor with particular attention to kidney function and once started it is usually lifelong. If blood pressure is very high – 'malignant hypertension' – and causing complications admission to hospital may be required.

Hypotension (low blood pressure)

When compared to the general population, this is a very common condition in adults with Down syndrome. As for hypertension, the BP must be measured on several occasions before it can be declared abnormally low. Hypertension for adults with Down syndrome is a systolic BP less than 90mmHg and/or a diastolic BP less than 50mmHg.

Causes: In the vast majority of people no cause is found, but dehydration, the side-effects of medication, hypothyroidism, and acute anxiety attacks are causes to look out for.

Symptoms and signs: Often there are no symptoms, but severe hypotension can present with dizziness when sitting or standing up, fainting episodes, headaches, and shortness of breath, dizziness or confusion.

Investigations: Initially there is a need to measure the BP on several occasions to confirm a persistently low level. Blood tests will be necessary to investigate for a possible underlying cause. It is also useful to measure the BP when standing and when sitting.

Complications: Though not directly due to hypotension, falls and loss of consciousness can lead to secondary injuries.

Treatment and prevention: As for hypertension, regular BP checks should be undertaken for all adults with Down syndrome, but in particular for those with a previous low level. The person should maintain good fluid intake, increase salt intake and avoid situations that are known to cause hypotension eg standing up too quickly, watching scary movies and rooms over-heated. Medication can be prescribed to increase blood pressure, but should be used with caution.

Heart problems

The heart is basically a pump made of muscle ensuring that blood is moved around the body. There are four chambers, two at the top (left and right atrium) and two at the bottom (left and right ventricles). Muscle walls (septa) and valves keep the chambers separate (Figure 7). Blood from the body collects in the right atrium, enters the right ventricle, is pumped to the lungs to collect oxygen, returns to the left atrium, enters the left ventricle and is pumped to the body, only to later return again to the right atrium. Problems can occur with a 'hole' being present in the muscle wall dividing the chambers (see specific heart lesions below), in the function of the heart valves, in the muscle of the heart or with the vessels returning or taking blood away from the heart.

Causes: (See specific heart lesions below). The vast majority of abnormalities are present at birth and should be detected at birth as part of a health screening programme. Some problems can present in later life because of the deterioration of childhood abnormalities or as part of weakness in the muscles of the heart valves or following untreated hypertension (above).

Symptoms and signs/complications: Valve defects and 'holes' in the heart impair the efficiency of the heart by causing blood to flow in a different direction. If left untreated this leads to different chambers working harder than expected which can in turn lead to heart failure (below) or lung disease (Chapter 7). The greater the defect, the greater the stress experienced by the heart.

Investigations: The severity and type of heart problem needs to be detected. Tests to detect any damage to the heart or lungs include blood tests, a chest x-ray, electrocardiography (ECG, the assessment of the electrical activity of the heart) and an echocardiography (ultrasound of the heart).

Treatment and prevention: Routine screening for heart problems should be undertaken. Early diagnosis and management is essential for future good health and long-life. Treatment will depend on the cause and the severity of any problem. A combination of different treatments may be used; medication, oxygen and surgery. Different drugs can be prescribed; diuretics (to reduce fluid overload), digoxin (to help the heart beat stronger), anti-hypertensives (to reduce blood pressure). Supplemental oxygen can help those who are cyanotic and have severe heart and lung disease. A heart transplant can be considered.

Figure 7 **Structure of the heart**

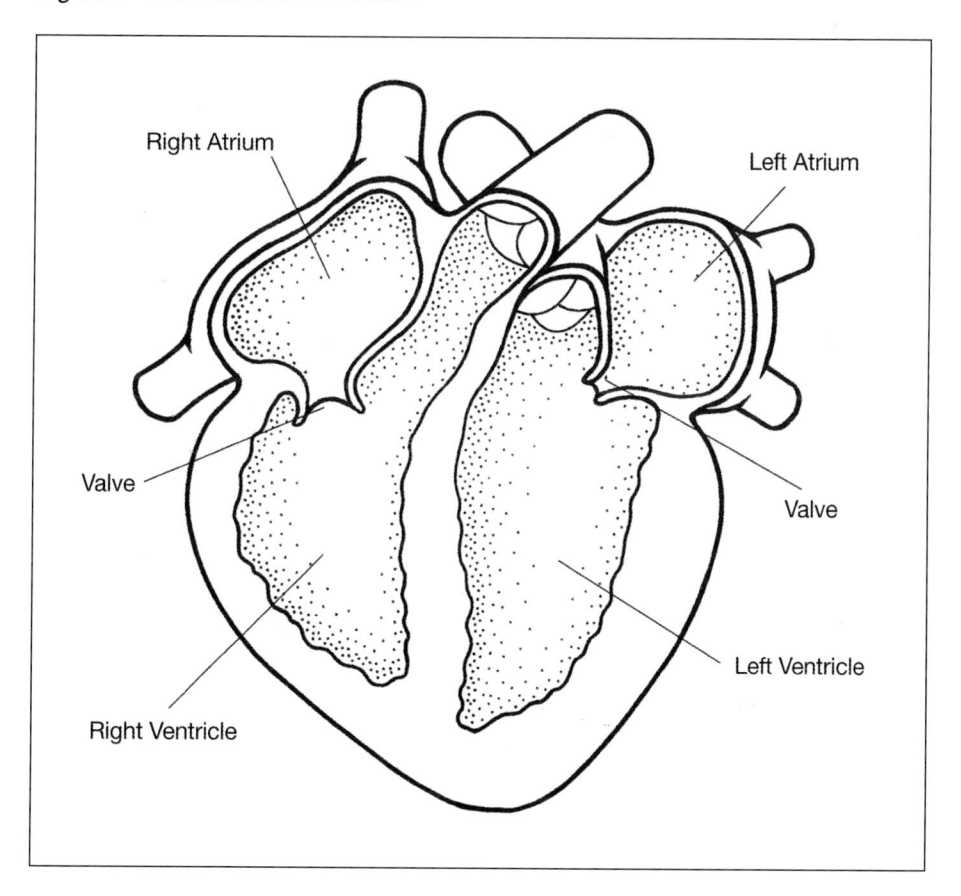

Specific heart lesions

Virtually all heart lesions in people with Down syndrome become apparent at or soon after birth. They should all be detected and treated if necessary during early childhood. However such problems can persist into adulthood or occur when a child with Down syndrome becomes an adult (eg mitral valve prolapsed). **Antibiotic cover must be given to any person with Down syndrome who is known to have a heart lesion and is about to undergo treatment which may lead to bacteria entering the bloodstream (see endocarditis below).**

Ventricular septal defect (VSD): This is a 'hole' in the muscle wall separating the two ventricles, which occurs in approximately 30% of all heart defects. A VSD results in blood flow from the left ventricle to the right ventricle. This can lead to high blood pressure in the blood vessels to the lungs. A VSD can occasionally be part of a condition called 'tetralogy of Fallot' (see below). Small VSDs may close spontaneously and cause no problems. Larger defects or those that lead to symptoms will need surgical closure.

Atrial septal defect (ASD): This is associated with blood flow from the left atrium to the right atrium. Usually an ASD does not lead to significant problems, but individuals can be prone to chest infections, breathlessness, tiredness, palpitations and an abnormal heart beat. The occurrence of a VSD and an ASD together is termed 'atrioventricular septal defect (AVSD)' and is quite common in people with Down syndrome. Small defects may close spontaneously or cause no significant problem, but larger defects will need surgical intervention to close the defect.

Patent ductus arteriosus: This condition occurs in approximately 5-10% of heart defects. The ductus arteriosus is a blood vessel near the heart which normally closes within 48 hours after birth, but if closure does not occur it remains open ('patent'). Often it can be a large opening and be associated with other defects. If untreated it can result in blood from the main blood vessel taking blood away from the heart to the rest of the body (aorta) flowing into the main artery of the lungs and leading to hypertension in the vessels of the lungs. If this is causing problems it will need surgical intervention.

Aortic coarctation: This is a narrowing of the main blood vessel (the aorta) taking blood away from the heart. Symptoms are often absent, but hypertension in the upper part of the body can develop. It may require surgical intervention.

Mitral valve prolapse (MVP): This is a malfunction of the mitral valve (the valve that controls blood flow from the left atrium to the left ventricle). It may develop in later life. Mild MVP is common in about one-third of people with Down syndrome. Mitral valve prolapse may be associated with an ASD (above) and keratoconus (Chapter 4). Usually heart lesions are detected by the presence of a heart murmur or when they lead to heart failure (below). Screening for MVP by echocardiography (ultrasound of the heart to produce moving images) has been recommended by some doctors. If severe, surgical intervention will be necessary.

Tetralogy of Fallot: A group of heart lesions present at birth. They should be detected at birth or early childhood, but problems may persist into adulthood.

Causes: These include a VSD (see heart lesions above), narrowing of blood vessel to lungs, right ventricle enlargement and abnormalities of the aorta (main blood vessel taking blood away from the heart), leading to mixing of blood within the heart.

Symptoms and signs: Common symptoms include tiredness, cyanosis (morbid bluish decolourisation of skin and lips), squatting after exercise and the presence of several heart murmurs.

Investigations: (See heart problems above).

Complications: The condition can result in heart failure (see below), polycythemia (Chapter 14) and can be life threatening.

Treatment and prevention: After exercise the squatting position can help. Any resulting heart failure and fevers must be treated promptly. Adults with Down syndrome with this condition should have been treated in childhood with surgery to close and correct defects.

Heart failure

A condition where the heart is unable to work properly in pumping blood around the body, resulting in inadequate oxygen supply to tissues.

Causes: There are a number of causes of heart failure, but the most important ones for adults with Down syndrome are heart lesions (above), thyroid disorders (Chapter 14) and lung disease (Chapter 7). Heart failure may affect only the left side of the heart, only the right side or both sides (called 'congestive heart failure').

Symptoms and signs: Symptoms are mainly caused by fluid accumulating either in the lungs or peripheral tissues and may not be present until permanent damage has occurred. Coughing, fast heart beat, sweating, paleness, chest infections, fainting, fatigue, breathlessness, chest deformities and an enlarged heart may be detected. On examination there may be a heart murmur, weight gain, swollen legs, laboured breathing with excessive chest movement and a rapid heart rate. Fluid in the lungs may be present. An enlarged liver or polycythemia (an increase in the amount of haemoglobin in the blood; see Chapter 14) may be seen.

Investigations: (See heart problems above).

Complications: If untreated the condition is life threatening.

Treatment: Medication (eg diuretics, beta-blockers, and digoxin) may be given to treat the heart failure. Surgery may be considered for replacement of defective valves or correction of heart lesions. Antibiotic cover when going to the dentist or going for any kind of surgery is necessary to prevent any infection which may get into the bloodstream settling in the heart (see endocarditis below). Drugs to stimulate the heart and improve muscle function may be used in a hospital setting. Depending on the cause, a heart transplant may be considered.

Endocarditis

An infection of the lining of the heart, usually of the heart valves or at the site of a heart lesion.

Causes: Usually caused by bacteria, from the mouth or from the urinary system at the time of dental treatment or after a urinary infection or procedure, which can enter the blood circulation and then settle on susceptible heart abnormalities.

Symptoms and signs: These include fever, night sweats, weight loss, weakness, changing murmur, skin lesions, microscopic signs of blood in urine, attacks of abdominal pain (due to clots dislodged from the heart) and heart failure (see above).

Investigations: These include blood screening for anaemia or evidence of inflammation, urine screening for blood being passed in urine, repeated blood analysis to isolate infective organism, echocardiogram (recording of an ultrasound of the heart) and chest x-ray to detect damage to heart.

Complications: Endocarditis can lead to heart failure; clumps of bacteria can be dislodged from the heart and can block off the blood supply to other organs eg kidneys, spleen, lungs. Infected clots lodged in the brain can cause brain abscesses. This can be a fatal condition.

Treatment and prevention: Any underlying infection must be treated with antibiotics. Surgery may be necessary if damage has occurred to any heart valve. **Treatment with antibiotics one hour before any procedure which may lead to bacteria entering the bloodstream (eg dental treatment) in individuals with a heart defect is essential to prevent endocarditis.** Good dental hygiene is important (Chapter 12).

Eisenmenger complex
This is a disorder affecting the heart and lungs together due to a long-standing heart lesion (ASD, VSD or patent ductus arteriosus see above).

Cause: The presence of a heart lesion where blood flows from left to right can lead over time to damage to the blood vessels in the lungs. This can increase resistance to blood passing through the lungs which in turn leads to increased work put on the right side of the heart. A higher pressure on the right side means blood may flow from right to left. Meaning blood containing little oxygen is being pumped around the body causing hypoxia (low oxygen levels).

Symptoms and signs: Frequent symptoms include a morbid blueness of the skin and lips (cyanosis), recurrent chest infections, breathlessness, tiredness, chest pain, swollen legs, fainting and headaches.

Investigations: Investigations undertaken to confirm the disorder and to detect degree of damage present include an echocardiogram (recording of an ultra-sound of the heart), a chest x-ray, cardiac catheterization (insertion of a fine tube into a blood vessel in the groin and passed into the heart) and blood tests to measure the thickness of blood and the blood haemoglobin concentration.

Complications: The condition can result in permanent heart damage, heart failure, polycythemia (Chapter 14).

Treatment: Blood may need to be removed (similar to what is done when giving a blood donation) to reduce its thickness and to reduce stress on the heart. Regular monitoring by a heart specialist doctor to prevent future lung damage is important. A heart and lung transplantation may be required if the condition becomes severe.

Coronary artery disease

Diseases of the blood vessels that supply oxygen to the heart are less common in adults with Down syndrome than the general population, but are, however, still a leading cause of death.

Causes: The blood vessels become narrowed due to the formation of 'sticky' fat deposits on the inside of the vessels (atherosclerosis). Obesity, diabetes mellitus, prematurity, high cholesterol levels, smoking and family history are contributing factors.

Symptoms and signs: Depending on the resulting damage to the heart, these might include the severe chest pain of a heart attack, breathlessness, chest pain during exercise, tiredness, swollen legs of heart failure (above) or fainting due to abnormal heart rhythm.

Investigations: These are undertaken to confirm the severity of vessel blockage and any associated complications and include an echocardiogram (recording of an ultra-sound of the heart), a chest x-ray, cardiac catheterisation (insertion of a fine tube into a blood vessel in the groin and passed into the heart).

Complications: Problems can include myocardial infarction (heart attack), angina, heart failure or abnormal rhythm of the heart.

Treatment and prevention: It is important to reduce risk factors for coronary artery disease such as smoking, diabetes mellitus, obesity, hypertension and high cholesterol levels, and to provide medical care for heart attack, heart failure, arrhythmia. In an acute heart attack, if appropriate, certain patients may undergo PCI (percutaneous intervention) where any blockage is removed. An angiogram may be carried out in those who are at high risk of a heart attack and if blockages are seen they can be removed or a stent inserted. Coronary artery bypass surgery where a blood vessel from elsewhere in the body is used to 'bypass' the blockage is being used less except for those with multiple blockages. The use of cholesterol reducing medication (eg statins) for people with Down syndrome is still controversial.

Varicose veins

A condition where the veins close to the surface of the skin are enlarged.

Causes: Varicose veins are due to the blood vessels losing their elasticity.

Symptoms and signs: No symptoms may be present, but there can occasionally be aches, swelling of the legs and veins which look like 'worms'.

Investigations: Varicose veins are usually diagnosed by appearance. A scan of the varicose veins is sometimes undertaken.

Complications: There may be discolouration of the skin or leg ulcers.

Treatment and prevention: **Varicose veins do not need treatment unless causing significant pain or to treat ulcers.** The person should avoid standing or sitting for long periods and in one place. Moving around and elevating legs to hip level can reduce severity. Salt intake should be limited to reduce any swelling. Support stockings are now widely available to provide compression for the legs. Veins can be removed in an operation called a phlebectomy. Newer treatments include 'sclerotherapy' (a chemical is injected into the varicose veins), laser or ablation therapy or the veins 'stripped' out of the leg.

Chapter 7

Respiratory system

Breathing and airway related problems can vary from minor but irritating, colds to life threatening respiratory failure. Chest infections and breathing problems are more common in people with Down syndrome than the general population due to the underlying differences in structure and function of the airways. Frequent, but minor conditions are discussed here as well as the less common, but more serious health problems. It must be borne in mind that chest infections still remain a major cause of death in adults with Down syndrome. **If breathing or swallowing is difficult and symptoms are severe or prolonged then a medical opinion should always be sought**.

Common cold

Causes: This is usually due to a viral infection which can be highly infectious in the early stages. The common cold is spread by direct contact with infected secretions from contaminated surfaces or by inhaling the airborne virus after individuals sneeze or cough. Person-to-person spread can occur when an individual who has a cold blows or touches their nose and then touches others or objects later touched by others. A cold virus can live on everyday objects such as pens, books, telephones, and cups for several hours and can thus be acquired from contact with these objects. Colds are more common in the winter months.

Symptoms and signs: Common symptoms include a slight temperature, tiredness, sneezing, sore nose and throat, watering eyes, headache and nasal discharge (watery initially, but later thick and 'green').

Investigations: Usually none are needed, but if persistent, blood tests may be required to detect evidence of infection and a sputum analysis for evidence and type of infection and to investigate the person's immune system.

Complications: The infection can spread to other areas, in particular the upper airways, sinuses, lungs and middle ear. A cold can result in bronchitis, asthma, sinusitis and ear infections.

Treatment and prevention: Most colds usually clear within one week. A warm humid room, regular paracetamol for aches and pains, bed rest, plenty of fluid intake, continuing to eat some food and a steam inhalation can be of benefit.

If a cold persists, if symptoms are severe, or a secondary bacterial infection occurs, antibiotics may be required. Over-the-counter remedies usually include a painkiller, decongestant and an antihistamine (a drug that blocks the action of histamine which is involved in producing an allergic reaction eg astemizole and terfenadine may relieve the symptoms). There is no definite prevention known, but large quantities of Vitamin C may help. Basic hygiene, ie regular hand washing when in contact with people who are unwell, sneezing into tissues and disposing of them appropriately can limit the spread of infection.

Nosebleed (epistaxis)
Bleeding usually from the blood vessels on the nasal septum.

Causes: Most nosebleeds have no particular cause but they are commonly due to picking of the nose or blowing of the nose. They can be due to hypertension (Chapter 6), inflammation of the nasal cavity, a general bleeding disorder or prescribed blood-thinning medicines (anticoagulants).

Symptoms and signs: As well as bleeding there may be other symptoms associated with an underlying cause.

Investigations: Usually none is required. If nosebleeds persist, underlying causes such as hypertension or blood clotting problems should be investigated.

Complications: These are rare, but shock or anaemia can develop if the bleed is longstanding or heavy.

Treatment and prevention: The person should be treated in a sitting up position, a firm pressure applied to the nostrils for at least 10 minutes using the finger and thumb. An ice-pack can be applied to the bridge of the nose. If bleeding persists the person will need medical attention where anaesthetic spray can be applied to constrict blood vessels and insertion of a nasal pack to stop further bleeding. Cauterising may be used to stop the bleeding. This involves sealing the bleeding area by using a low level of heat or a tiny dab of silver nitrate (which can be painful). The person should avoid picking the nose and blowing it hard if it's blocked due to a cold or hay fever.

Sore throat (pharyngitis)
An inflammation of the throat between the tonsils and the upper part of the windpipe.

Causes: Often this is part of a common cold (above) and caused usually by a virus, but sometimes it can be bacterial. No known cause may be identified.

Symptoms and signs: As well as a sore throat, the top of the mouth can be reddened and tonsils inflamed and swollen. There may be discomfort on swallowing, slight fever or earache. The lymph nodes in the neck may be enlarged.

Investigations: (See common cold above). If the soreness persists a throat swab can be taken to isolate the cause of the inflammation.

Complications: The inflammation can occasionally spread to involve other parts of the airways. Epidemics can occur.

Treatment: The disease is self-limiting and symptomatic relief is usually all that is required. Gargling with warm salt water, avoiding lying flat and use of painkillers can help. Antiseptic lozenges and sprays can make things worse. The person should keep hydrated and avoid food and drinks that irritate the throat. For severe or persistent tonsillitis antibiotics may be required. The GP should be consulted if there is a persistent high temperature above 38C (100.4F) which is not reduced by medication, if symptoms do not improve after two weeks, if there are frequent sore throats that do not respond to painkillers, such as paracetamol, ibuprofen or aspirin or if there is a spread of the infection to the airways and lungs.

Hayfever (seasonal rhinitis)

Causes: Commonly an allergic reaction usually to tree or grass pollen or mould spores. More common in young adults, in people with asthma and/or eczema and usually worst in June and July when pollen counts are higher.

Symptoms and signs: These include nasal irritation, sneezing, watery runny nose, itching of eyes or top of mouth or ear. If hayfever is severe it can cause loss of the sense of smell, facial pain (caused by blocked sinuses), sweats and headaches.

Investigations: Detailed history is often all that is needed to make a diagnosis. Skin-prick testing for allergies and an assessment of immune status with blood tests can be undertaken.

Complications: Usually none but breathing and feeding difficulties, sleep disturbance and ear infections can occur. Sinusitis (see below) is possible and the condition can impact on day-to-day activities.

Treatment and prevention: The best is to avoid or reduce contact with allergen. Antihistamines (group of drugs that block the action of histamine which is necessary to produce an allergic reaction eg loratadine, cetirizine) can be prescribed or purchased at the pharmacists. Decongestants, steroids, anti-inflammatory drugs may also be given. Older antihistamines are associated with sedation.

Constant runny nose (perennial rhinitis)
A constant nasal discharge throughout the year.

Causes: There are allergic types (to house dust mite, pollen grains, domestic animals, moulds) and non-allergic types.

Symptoms and signs: These include sneezing, watery runny nose, nasal blockage, loss of smell and taste and sinusitis.

Investigation/complications/treatment and prevention: (see hayfever above).

Enlarged adenoids
Swollen lymph glands found at the back of the nose. These glands are present to fight infections.

Causes: Caused by a viral or bacterial infection.

Symptoms and signs: These include snoring, chronic discharge from nose, cough.

Complications: Enlarged adenoids can lead to ear infections, 'glue ear' (Chapter 5), obstructive sleep apnoea.

Treatment: Any discharge from the nose should be cleared with steam inhalation and if necessary a course of antibiotics. For recurrent cases surgical removal of the adenoids (adenoidectomy) may be necessary.

Sinusitis
An inflammation of the sinuses (air cavities found near the nose within the skull).

Causes: Usually following a nasal infection, less commonly from dental disease.

Symptoms and signs: These include increased nasal discharge, headaches, and tenderness over cheeks, feeling of fullness in the affected area, throbbing ache, loss of smell and a high temperature. The presence of a green/yellow nasal discharge suggests a bacterial infection.

Investigations: Usually none are required, but an x-ray examination of the sinuses can show evidence of the inflammation.

Complications: Breathing and feeding difficulties are possible and the condition can in rare cases lead to meningitis or the spread of infection into the blood.

Treatment: Persistent problems with clear drainage suggest a possible allergic reaction and antihistamines, painkillers or decongestants may be of benefit. Steam drainage can be helpful along with warm face packs over cheeks. The person should keep well hydrated. A green-yellow discharge would suggest the need for antibiotics. Surgical drainage is occasionally considered.

Asthma

Contraction of the muscles of the airways and an inflammation of the small airways making breathing difficult; secondary to narrowing of the airways.

Causes: There can be a history of asthma in the family but often no cause is found. It can be due to allergies, eg pollen, house dust, animal fur or feathers, or to atmospheric pollution, smoke, drugs, infections, emotional upsets or exercise. Asthma usually starts in childhood and can clear with increasing age.

Symptoms and signs: The person has recurrent attacks of wheezing, shortness of breath, cough, tightness in the chest, a fast heart rate, it is often worse at night. In severe attacks breathing can be very difficult with considerable distress, anxiety and episodes of cyanosis when the lips become 'blue'.

Investigations: These may not be necessary initially, but in order to monitor how well the lungs are functioning a 'peak flow reading' is taken regularly. This involves the person blowing hard and fast into a peak flow meter. Blood and sputum tests can be undertaken to detect any infection. A chest x-ray can detect any damage to lungs. An allergen provocation test may be considered to find the allergy if one is suspected.

Complications: There can be difficulty sleeping (due to persistent cough) poor attendance at work, recurrent chest infections. Asthma can result in severe breathing difficulty (status asthmaticus), collapsed lung or respiratory failure. If untreated a severe attack can be life threatening.

Treatment and prevention: A stepwise regime is recommended. If the condition is mild, the person is given a 'reliever' inhaler (salbutamol) to use when the chest feels tight. If this inhaler is being used frequently or the person has moderate breathing difficulties 'preventer' inhalers can be used (inhaled steroid/inhaled beta-2 agonist). Once optimised on these inhalers, oral tablets (monteleukast/steroids) can be used. Once symptom control is achieved the individual can 'step down the ladder'. Further information about the stepwise approach is available at http://bit.ly/1eMCAYv. In chronic management, patient education and inhaler technique is vital. A spacer device is often given to younger people. For further information see http://bit.ly/1fVWLQd.

In an acute attack, more active medication is given, such as nebulisers, antibiotics and a short course of steroids. Recurrent attacks should be investigated for other underlying problems, eg foreign body in airways, immune deficiency and difficulty in administration of medication. Asthma can be a medical emergency. **If there is severe cyanosis or severe breathing problems request emergency paramedic help early as the person can deteriorate rapidly.**

Bronchitis
An inflammation of the airways to the lungs.

Causes: Bronchitis is often viral, but can be complicated by a bacterial infection. Smoking and air pollutants can predispose the person to infections.

Acute symptoms and signs: These include an irritating unproductive cough, discomfort and tightness in chest, wheezing and shortness of breath, headaches, slight fever, blocked nose and sinuses, a cough which is later productive of yellow or green sputum, mild fever.

Chronic symptoms and signs: The person experiences several episodes of coughing with the production of sputum, wheezing and breathlessness. Frequent infections and exacerbation can occur in poor weather.

Investigations: An assessment of lung function with peak flow meters can be undertaken, a chest x-ray to show any infection and sputum analysis for evidence of infection. If necessary, blood tests can be done to measure the amount of oxygen and carbon dioxide in the bloodstream.

Complications: Bronchitis can occasionally lead to pneumonia (below) or heart failure (Chapter 6).

Treatment and prevention: The person should avoid smoking (active and passive) and air pollutants. The inhalation of steam and drinking plenty of fluids can help. Medication to improve breathing (bronchodilators, eg Ventolin, steroids and anti-inflammatory agents) and antibiotics for any infection may be prescribed. Physiotherapy and oxygen can be given to improve lung function.

Influenza
A viral infection of the airways which can affect adults with Down syndrome more seriously than adults in the general population due to their immune system dysfunction. Highly infectious.

Causes: Caused by a particular type of influenza virus which is often associated with local milder outbreaks. However worldwide epidemics can occur. The virus can be spread by the inhalation of infected droplets sneezed or coughed into the air. There are three types of virus: A, B, and C.

Symptoms and signs: The incubation period is 1-3 days and symptoms include sudden fever, shivering and shaking in limbs, severe headache, soreness of throat and persistent dry cough, muscle ache, fatigue and loss of appetite. Getting back to normal activities is usually achieved gradually. Secondary bacterial infections can occur.

Investigations: Usually none is necessary, body response to virus can be measured by means of a blood test if required and a chest x-ray can rule out pneumonia.

Complications: Influenza can lead to pneumonia (below), sinusitis (above), middle ear infection (Chapter 5), dehydration, meningitis (infection in the brain and spinal cord) encephalitis (inflammation of the brain), and post-infection depression or deterioration in previously well controlled mental illness.

Treatment and prevention: (See common cold above). Antiviral medications (Tamiflu, Relenza) are available but should be started within 48 hours of onset of symptoms. A vaccine, or flu jab, is recommended for anyone with reduced immune function to prevent them getting the illness. Vaccines tend to be effective in 70% of cases, but are often short-lasting. A vaccine should not be given if the person is allergic to egg protein.

Pneumonia
An inflammation of the lungs usually due to an infection. More common in older adults and adults with Down syndrome who have reduced immunity and difficulties in swallowing (leading to increased aspiration).

Causes: Pneumonia is usually due to a viral or bacterial infection, but can be a fungal or parasite infection.

Symptoms and signs: Common symptoms include a high temperature, chest pain, dry cough, rusty-coloured sputum, fast breathing and difficulty in breathing, rapid heartbeat, feeling weak, mental confusion and irritability.

Investigations: A chest x-ray will be required, as well as a sputum analysis to identify the infective agent and a blood screen for evidence and type of infection. Blood oxygen level tests may be necessary in severe cases.

Complications: Pneumonia can lead to an inflammation around the lungs (pleurisy), fluid collection or an abscess (collection of pus) in the lungs, a collapsed lung, respiratory failure and spread of infection into the bloodstream (septicaemia). If not treated pneumonia can in some cases be life threatening.

Treatment and prevention: The condition can usually be managed at home, but may require hospitalisation. Plenty of fluids (oral/intravenous), physiotherapy to chest and analgesia (paracetamol, aspirin) are required. Hospital care with lung ventilation will be required in severe cases where there is low oxygen in the blood. Anti-infection drugs can be given. Knowing the cause of the pneumonia will aid prevention. For example if there are problems with swallowing, advice can be given to reduce the risk of a recurrence. 'Pneumovax', an anti-pneumococcal vaccine, can be given to anyone over 50 years or with reduced immune function.

Obstructive sleep apnoea (OSA)

A condition in which the airway at the back of the throat is sucked closed when breathing in during sleep. The airflow is interrupted for usually more than 10 seconds.

Causes: Often no single factor is found. The condition is associated with poor muscle tone, small upper airways, frequent chest infections, obesity, hypothyroidism, enlarged tonsils or adenoids, nasal obstruction and drugs affecting respiration, eg sedatives and strong analgesia.

Symptoms and signs: These include loud snoring, daytime sleeping, restless sleep, morning headache, mouth breathing, nocturnal choking, poor concentration, irritability and behaviour changes.

Investigations: An abnormal night-time breathing pattern needs to be confirmed. Videotaping of night-time breathing is important. 'Oximetry-testing' is required to confirm the disorder. This is where the brain waves, blood oxygen levels, muscle tone and movement and other bodily signs are measured whilst the person sleeps.

Complications: OSA can cause hypertension or heart failure (Chapter 6), a stroke or lung disease.

Treatment and prevention: Any underlying factors (eg lose weight), need to be treated. Sedating drugs and sleep deprivation should be avoided. Antidepressants (group of drugs used to treat depression eg amitripytline, fluoxetine) can help in milder cases. The person may need what is termed 'continuous positive airway pressure' which involves giving oxygen and air under pressure via a tightly fitted face mask. A tonsillectomy and/or an adenoidectomy (surgical removal of the adenoids),maxillomandibular advancement (a surgical procedure which moves the jaw top [maxilla] and bottom [mandible] forward), may be necessary.

Chapter 8

Digestive system

Digestive problems can be present at birth and persist throughout the lifetime of a person with Down syndrome or they can develop later during adulthood. Problems may arise with the structure or the function of the gut (Figure 8). Family members and paid support staff need to be vigilant for any symptoms or signs suggesting an underlying serious problem such as blood in stools, marked weight loss, severe abdominal pain. Minor as well as the more serious health problems that can occur in adults with Down syndrome, and which are associated with the digestive system, are discussed in this chapter. **Persistent, severe symptoms or deterioration in health necessitate a medical assessment.**

Figure 8 **Digestive system**

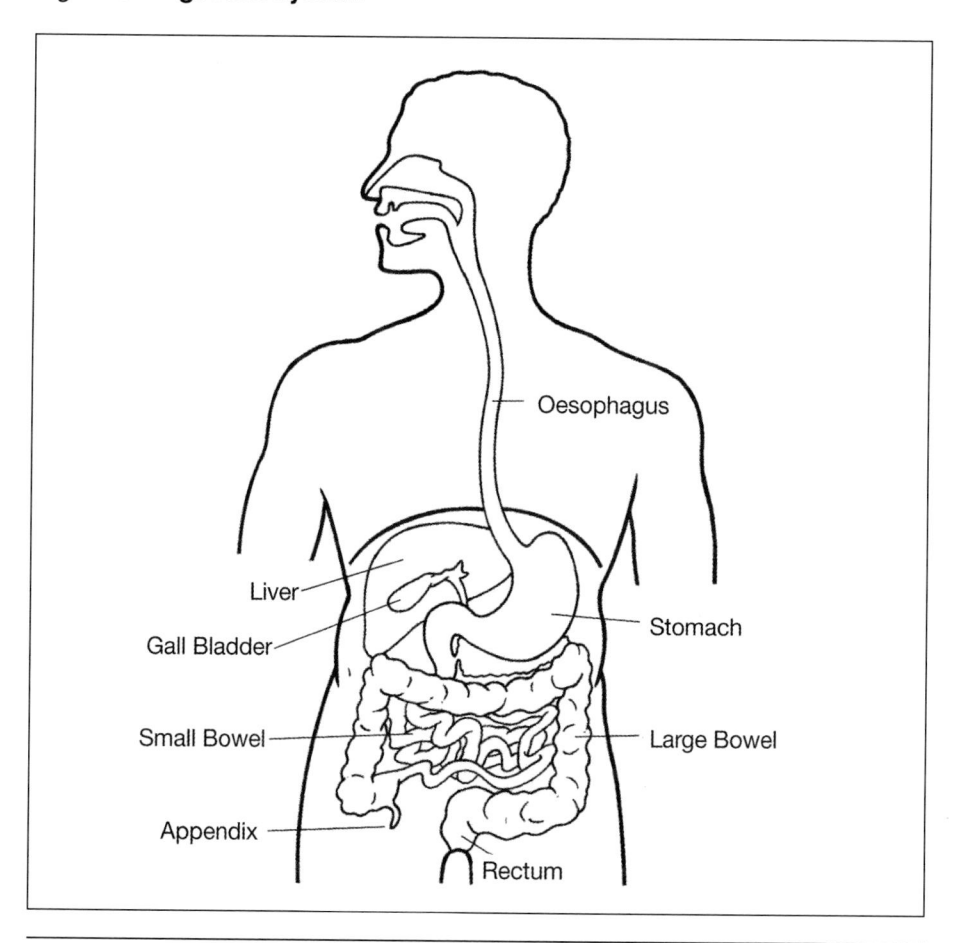

Choking

Causes: An obstruction of the throat usually with food, drink or swallowing an object such as a peanut or bead leading to difficulty in breathing. Can be due to throat inflammation.

Symptoms and signs: The person may look 'blue', be speechless and in distress. Breathing, if still possible, is laboured, producing gasping. The person cannot speak or cry out, or has great difficulty and limited ability to do so. They desperately clutch the throat or mouth. If breathing is not restored, then they will become unconscious.

Complications: If not managed immediately choking can lead to death.

Treatment: Different procedures are used to increase abdominal pressure to enable any object in the throat to be expelled out of the mouth. The main procedures are encouraging the person to cough, several back slaps (heel of the hand on the upper back) and abdominal thrusts, also known by the proprietary name the Heimlich Manoeuvre. This manoeuvre involves a first aider standing behind the person and using their hands to exert pressure on the bottom of the diaphragm. This compresses the lungs and exerts an upwards pressure on any object lodged in the throat, hopefully expelling it. **Emergency help should be summoned if first aid is unsuccessful.**

There is more information about the Heimlich manoeuvre and other first aid skills in the book Bradley, A (2013) *Health and Safety for Learning Disability Workers* (Appendix D).

Vomiting
Vomiting is the body's way of trying to get rid of harmful substances from the stomach, or is a reaction to something that has irritated the gut. It can be associated with wanting to vomit (nausea) and effort to vomit (retching).

Causes: Common reasons include pregnancy, travel sickness, ear or urine infection, emotional upset, general illness or side-effects of medication.
The more important medical causes related to the digestive system include constipation, bowel obstruction, food poisoning, gastroenteritis, reflux, coeliac disease (below) appendicitis and an ulcer. In these conditions vomiting is usually associated with abdominal pain. Other causes to consider include migraine, meningitis, diabetes, metabolic problems, over-eating and self-induced vomiting.

Symptoms and signs: Looking pale and sweating can occur prior to vomiting. Blood or 'coffee ground' vomit can be a sign of bleeding in the gastro-intestinal tract. Other features are associated with the underlying cause.

Investigations: These depend on the likely cause, but can include blood and urine tests for infection, x-ray examination, ultrasound and an endoscopy (passing of flexible tube through the mouth down into the digestive system to view inside) to detect any abdominal problem.

Complications: If vomiting is persistent it can lead to an imbalance in body electrolytes (specific chemicals in the blood required for good health), dehydration or lung inflammation due to substances going into the lungs. Repeated or profuse vomiting may cause erosions or a tear in the oesophagus. Specific complications may be associated with a given cause.

Treatment: Treatment depends on the cause. If the cause is obvious and not serious, vomiting just needs to be monitored and fluids given for rehydration. No food or drink should be taken during episodes of vomiting if a more serious cause is suspected. Drugs (called anti-emetics, eg metoclopramide) can be given to stop the vomiting. The underlying cause, eg infection, needs to be treated with antibiotics, constipation with laxatives; medication must be stopped if the vomiting is a side effect. If vomiting is severe, lasts more than 24 hours or blood is present seek medical advice.

Eating problems
Eating problems are common in people with Down syndrome.

Causes: These can relate to the person's social or emotional situation, be personality or situation related, or associated with a physical or mental health disorder or condition, eg obsessive disorder, autism (Chapter 15).

Symptoms and signs: Eating problems can include refusal to eat textured food, chewing difficulties, eating only specific foods, being slow to finish a meal, throwing food away and hoarding food.

Investigations: Where there have been no previous problems with eating, an underlying physical or emotional cause such as a problem with swallowing (dysphagia), constipation, depression, an obsessive disorder (Chapter 15) should be investigated. The person's weight should be monitored.
An assessment from a speech and language therapist who specialises in dysphagia, or a dietician or psychologist may be required.

Complications: Weight loss (below), behavioural changes, constipation and nutritional deficiency (Chapter 2) can occur. Family members and paid support staff can find it stressful to support the person when they have problems with eating.

Treatment and prevention: Education about appropriate food intake, making mealtimes distinct and inviting, encouraging eating with attention and/or special favourite foods after completion of meals should be recommended. Training in cooking skills, dieting and exercise can have considerable benefit. For adults with behavioural changes early intervention from a dietician or psychologist can be beneficial. If an underlying mental health disorder is present (depression, obsessive disorder – see Chapter 15) then treatment by a psychiatrist may be necessary. Support for family members and paid staff is important as well as ongoing monitoring of the person's weight and calorie intake. Supplementation with megavitamin therapy is not recommended.

Weight loss

It is important to compare the weight of a person with Down syndrome not only to people in the general population, but also to that of other people with Down syndrome of the same age and sex (Chapter 2). It is also important to compare the present weight to previous weight measurements.

Causes: The level of exercise and calorie intake will affect weight loss. Dieting and refusal to eat are intentional causes. Unintentional weight loss can be due to reduced appetite as a result of abdominal discomfort, physical or mental ill-health, such as depression or dementia (Chapter 15). Weight loss with a good appetite still present can be due to hyperthyroidism or diabetes (Chapter 14), an infection, abdominal disease and rarely, cancer.

Symptoms and signs: Weight loss other than by weighing may be observed by clothes becoming loose, comments from others about the person looking physically or emotionally unwell. Other symptoms may be associated with a particular cause.

Investigations: Investigation depends on cause and severity. A general medical investigation may be necessary to determine any underlying physical or psychological cause. Tests include urine or stool analysis, blood screen for inflammation or infection, endoscopic examination (means of looking directly into digestive system by using a flexible tube), x-ray and ultrasound assessments (a procedure where sound waves are transmitted to the body and the reflection (echo) is detected using detectors, the echoes are converted by a computer to pictures).

Complications: Usually there are no complications unless there is severe and sudden weight loss leading to malnutrition, muscle wasting. Secondary problems may be associated with the underlying cause.

Treatment and prevention: Any underlying cause should be treated, calorie intake increased and exercise reduced. Advice and support from a dietician may be necessary. If refeeding occurs after a prolonged period of starvation, careful attention must be paid to regular blood tests so that the person concerned does not develop 'refeeding syndrome' (a condition in which metabolic disturbances occur after a period of severe malnutrition or starvation and which requires medical support).

Abdominal pain

Causes: Abdominal pain can be related to emotional upset, it may be part of a general illness or caused by a local abdominal problem. When due to gastrointestinal problems common causes include constipation (below), overeating and stomach irritation. It can also be because of some other more serious abdominal problem (eg blockage to bowels – see below). It may be a common illness such as irritable bowel syndrome (see below).

Symptoms and signs: Site, intensity, duration, character, aggravating and relieving factors and associated symptoms are important information relating to the pain. A central dull abdominal pain is usually due to stomach irritation (eg increased gastric acidity, peptic ulcer disease). Right upper abdomen pain can be due to gallbladder or biliary tract inflammation. Lower abdominal pain can be due to bladder infection, bowel problems or gynaecological problems. Some adults with Down syndrome may not be able to vocalise any discomfort, but present with emotional or behavioural changes.

Investigations: (See weight loss above).

Complications: Abdominal pain can lead to marked behaviour and/or emotional changes or other complications secondary to the underlying cause.

Treatment: Reassurance may be all that is required if the pain is mild. Recurrent attacks of mild pain may settle with simple painkillers, a milky drink, a hot-water bottle and bed rest. More serious causes will need specific management and if pain is severe or persistent the person will need a medical or surgical assessment.

Mouth ulcers
Mouth ulcers are painful round or oval sores that form in the mouth, often on the inside of the cheeks.

Causes: There may be no one particular cause, the cause may be unknown or the ulcer may be due to trauma, infection (eg herpes), or associated with bowel disease, nutritional deficiencies, or drug therapy.

Symptoms and signs: May mimic toothache (Chapter 12). Avoidance of contact with the ulcer when eating is common. Pain may be experienced on brushing the teeth near the ulcer.

Complications: Usually none.

Treatment and prevention: Most mouth ulcers clear up after a few days without any intervention. The person should use a soft toothbrush when brushing teeth and avoid eating hard foods, such as toast. Application to the ulcer of a gel containing chlorhexidine (eg Corsodyl) or steroids can temporarily relieve pain. Antimicrobial mouthwash can reduce organisms in the mouth that cause ulcers. A dentist should be consulted if the condition persists longer than two weeks or if there is no response to simple measures. Good gum and teeth hygiene can prevent recurrence.

Bowel obstruction
A blockage to the bowel preventing passage of contents along the full length of the bowel.

Causes: There are many possible causes, from a swallowed foreign body, problems in bowel motility, twisting of the bowel, growths in the bowel or compression of the bowel from the outside.

Symptoms and signs: These depend on the site of the obstruction, but generally include nausea and vomiting, abdominal pain, constipation, no passage of wind, colic and swelling of the abdomen. Behavioural or emotional changes can be the first sign of a physical problem.

Investigations: Common tests undertaken to find severity and cause include an x-ray examination, ultrasound of abdomen, blood screen for chemical imbalance, and an endoscopy (means of looking into the digestive system by using a flexible tube).

Complications: Complications are rare, but a rupture of the bowel can occur leading to peritonitis (inflammation of the lining of the abdomen).

Treatment: Bowel obstruction requires medical intervention. Treatment depends on the cause; for example, if an object has been swallowed, it will need to be removed, constipation will require either strong laxatives taken by mouth or a rectal enema. If simple measures fail the person may need admission to hospital for further treatment. This includes trying to reduce the abdominal distension with a tube (nasogastric tube) passed through the nose into the stomach to remove the build up of gas, replacement of fluids lost and surgery to remove the obstruction.

Constipation

The passage of small hard faeces infrequently and with difficulty. There is a wide normal variation of bowel habit (several times a day to twice a week/weekly). A change from normal habit is important to note. It is a common problem in people with Down syndrome because of low muscle tone, reduced mobility and selective diets.

Causes: These include inadequate fibre in the diet, reduced fluid intake, lack of regular daily habits, lack of physical activity, diet, hypothyroidism (Chapter 14), depression (Chapter 15), side-effects of drugs and bowel disease.

Symptoms and signs: Flatulence, bloating, abdominal pain, small hard stools and over-flow diarrhoea are common symptoms. Behavioural changes can occur. In epilepsy, constipation is possibly associated with deterioration.

Investigations: If constipation persists the person may require abdominal x-ray examinations and blood tests to exclude thyroid disease.

Complications: Bowel obstruction is possible (above).

Treatment and prevention: A high-fibre diet is beneficial, eg whole grain cereals, bran, raw fruits and vegetables, and adequate fluid intake. Prunes can act as a laxative. Active exercise can aid movement of stool through the bowel. Regular bowel habits and good toileting skills are important. Glycerol suppositories, laxatives and enemas can be prescribed, but prolonged use can impair normal functioning. Any underlying cause should be treated.

Diarrhoea

Frequently passed loose stools. There is a wide normal variation in bowel habit so a change from normal frequency is important. Watery large volume stools suggest a bowel infection (especially if bloody).

Causes: These include dietary causes, bowel infection, bowel disease, drugs, metabolic problems, faecal impaction and emotional problems.
Acute diarrhoea can occur for a few days, usually due to contaminated food or drink and settles without intervention. Chronic diarrhoea may be due to bowel disease, hyperthyroidism, irritable bowel disease or from side-effects of medication.

Symptoms and signs: These include loose motions, cramp-like abdominal pain, distress, restlessness, weight loss, blood in stools and associated fever.

Investigations: Further assessment may be required, including rectal examination, stool analysis to identify any infection, blood tests, x-ray examination or biopsy of the bowel.

Complications: Dehydration is possible and can present as drowsiness, unresponsiveness, glazed eyes, dry mouth and poor urine output. If severe dehydration occurs then hospital admission to rehydrate will be needed. Blood chemical imbalance can occur if diarrhoea is severe or prolonged.

Treatment: Fluid loss can be replaced initially with clear water with dissolved sugar and no solids given until diarrhoea ends. Food should be introduced gradually. Anti-diarrhoea drugs (group of drugs used to stop diarrhoea either by forming bulk, eg Kaolin mixture or reducing gut motility (eg codeine phosphate) can be of help but should be avoided in an infective cause. Any underlying cause should be treated.

Coeliac disease

Malabsorption syndrome. Usually diagnosed in childhood but can present at any age. More common in people with Down syndrome than the general population.

Causes: The body develops an allergy to 'gluten' protein found in wheat and cereal grains. The bowel wall becomes inflamed and the lining becomes flat, impairing absorption of foods and minerals.

Symptoms and signs: These include abnormal stools (diarrhoea, foul smelling), swollen abdomen, irritability, anaemia, tiredness, malaise, abdominal pain, muscle cramps, seizures, weight loss and vomiting.

Investigations: Blood tests are used for specific indicators of coeliac disease called 'anti-gliadin antibodies'. Antibodies are proteins produced by the body's immune system which help to neutralise infecting agents such as bacteria or viruses. Small bowel biopsy and blood tests for anaemia may be required.

Complications: Complications are usually seen in childhood (poor growth, failure to gain weight). If untreated and chronic the condition can lead to bowel cancer.

Treatment and prevention: The person needs a gluten-free diet and should avoid cereal wheat, rye, barley and possibly oats. Reintroduction of gluten will lead to the recurrence of symptoms. Maintenance to a strict diet is essential. Support and advice from a dietician is recommended. Iron replacement may be required initially.

Lactose intolerance
Inability to digest lactose, sugar found in cow's milk.

Causes: Individuals with lactose intolerance do not produce enough of the enzyme Lactase, which is necessary to breakdown lactose. The condition can develop in young adults following a gastroenteritis illness.

Symptoms and signs: These include a swollen abdomen, irritability, anaemia, tiredness, malaise, abdominal pain, muscle cramps, seizures and diarrhoea.

Investigations: Often none are needed, depending on the person's history. A lactose breath hydrogen test, which is simple and non-invasive, is performed after a short period of fasting (typically 8–12 hours). A base reading of hydrogen levels in the person's breath is taken first. They are then given a small amount of pure lactose and required to take several readings during the following 2-3 hours. If the level of hydrogen rises above 20 ppm (parts per million) over the lowest preceding value within the test period, the person is typically diagnosed as having lactose intolerance.

Complications: Lactose intolerance is usually seen in childhood (poor growth, failure to gain weight).

Treatment and prevention: The person needs a lactose-free diet and should avoid milk, cheese, ice-cream and prepared products containing lactulose. Milk treated with lactase and lactase tablets, and soy milk are now available. Calcium and vitamin D supplements may be necessary. Support and advice from a dietician is recommended.

Irritable bowel syndrome (IBS)
Intermittent pain and irregular bowel habit. Often repeated episodes.

Causes: There is no one cause, but IBS is reported to be associated with emotional distress leading to abnormal motility and spasms of the intestines.

Symptoms and signs: These include pain in the lower left abdomen which is relieved by opening bowels, alternating constipation and diarrhoea, abdominal distension and wind. A long history of such problems is usually reported.

Investigations: Investigations are rarely needed, but they can screen for a serious medical problem (see constipation and diarrhoea above). Tests are usually all normal.

Complications: IBS can cause secondary emotional distress.

Treatment and prevention: Reassurance and a high-fibre diet can benefit the majority of people. Anti-diarrhoea drugs can be prescribed depending on the predominant symptom. Anti-spasmodic medications reduce bowel spasms and therefore provide relief from cramping pains. Large meals, caffeine and fatty foods should be avoided. Occasionally low dose anti-depressants can be prescribed to reduce anxiety.

Gastroesophageal reflux disease (GORD)
Flow of acid from the stomach back up into the oesophagus. Often undiagnosed in people with Down syndrome, but can be quite common.

Causes: Obesity, over-eating, sleep apnoea, gallstones increase the risk of GORD but the cause is not always identified.

Symptoms and signs: These include heartburn, regurgitation of food, abdominal pain, hoarseness, cough, sore throat, aspiration, irritability, aggression, asthma, and erosion of teeth.

Investigations: Endoscopy (tube passed into mouth and down into stomach) and barium x-ray are used to investigate.

Complications: Inflammation of the oesophagus can occur and in severe cases scarring and constriction of the oesophagus. If prolonged, cells at the base of the oesophagus can become altered, 'Barrett's oesophagus' which requires closer follow up as these cells can become malignant.

Treatment and prevention: Simple measures such as not over-eating; sitting up after meals, looser trousers and other clothes can help considerably. Sleeping with upper body slightly raised can help where reflux is present on waking. Acidic fruit or juices, fatty foods, coffee, tea, onions and chocolate should be avoided. Peppermint has been shown to benefit some individuals. Medications such as antacids (aluminium hydroxide), H2 receptor blockers (eg cimetidine/ranitidine), proton-pump inhibitors (eg omeprazole, lansoprazole) can reduce acid erosion. Metoclopramide can be prescribed to help food to pass through the stomach.

Peptic ulcer disease
Irritation or erosions to the lining of the stomach or duodenum.

Causes: The commonest causes include reaction to nonsteroidal anti-inflammatory drug (NSAID) use, an organism called H. Pylori, alcohol and conditions which produce too much acid.

Symptoms and signs: These are similar to GORD (see above): central chest/upper abdominal discomfort, bloating, blood in vomit/coffee ground vomit and darkened stools.

Investigations: Endoscopy is the definitive investigation, a tube is placed into the stomach to look for an ulcer or the cause of the irritation. An H.Pylori breath test assesses the presence of this organism in the stomach. General blood tests are used to look for inflammation/infection.

Complications: There can be ongoing discomfort. If severe and prolonged, there may be massive blood loss or perforation of the stomach/duodenum.

Treatment and prevention: This depends on the cause. The main treatment is high dose proton-pump inhibitors (PPI) in an acute situation with prolonged lower dose PPI when symptoms are controlled. PPIs are a group of drugs whose main action is a pronounced and long-lasting reduction of gastric acid production. If the condition is due to the organism H.Pylori – irradiation using 'triple therapy' two different antibiotics and a PPI – is given for six weeks. If bleeding is seen at endoscopy the ulcers may then be treated.

Hepatitis

Inflammation of the liver which can be acute (sudden onset, jaundice, severe abdominal pain) or chronic (slow deterioration in liver function).

Causes: **Hepatitis A** is a viral infection passed usually by the faecal-oral route. The infected stool is touched by someone else (eg via toilet seat) who then touches their own mouth. **Hepatitis B** is a virus which can cause inflammation of the liver. A high frequency of chronic carriers (people with the virus, but showing no symptoms) has been found in residential care settings for people with a learning disability. Males are more infectious than females. Transmission appears to occur through skin or by contact of the inside of the mouth to blood and other bodily fluids. The greatest risk is from people who demonstrate biting and scratching behaviours. The **Hepatitis C** virus is most commonly transmitted via blood, in the past via blood transfusions. Blood is now tested before transfusion so this form of transmission now is rare. However people with Hepatitis C often develop chronic liver disease and this can cause an increased risk of liver cancer.

Symptoms and signs: Often none are present, but if present can include jaundice (yellow decolourisation of the skin due to liver disease), fever, loss of appetite, tenderness in right upper part of abdomen, nausea and vomiting, dark urine, pale stools and muscle aches.

Investigations: These include a blood test for antibodies (proteins produced by the body's immune system which help to neutralise infecting agents) to the virus, and liver function tests to assess the status of the liver. Other contacts need to be tested.

Complications: Occasionally hepatitis can result in liver failure or cause death.

Treatment and prevention: Good hygiene and hand washing is essential to prevent spread. Hepatitis A or B vaccination is important to reduce infection. Chronic Hepatitis B can be treated with Epivir, Hepsera and Hepatitis C with interferon. During the acute phase bed rest and a nourishing diet is recommended.

Chapter 9

Sexual health

The quality of genitourinary care for people with a learning disability (especially for women) remains poor. A number of studies have reported a low uptake of routine screening and health promotion activities amongst people with a learning disability. Among the reasons given is a lack of information suitable for people with a learning disability and the fact that some health providers do not understand the needs of people with a learning disability and therefore do not make the necessary reasonable adjustments to meet their needs.

This chapter deals with sexual health and the one that follows discusses issues relating to the urinary system.

People with Down syndrome, family members and paid staff can find information, guidance and counselling on menstrual, sexual and contraceptive issues from their GP, a local learning disability nurse as well as from FPA and other organisations (see Appendix E).

The opinion of a doctor or other suitable health care worker should be sought if the person with Down syndrome, family members or paid staff have any concerns about sexual health matters.

Sexual health issues for women

Most young women with Down syndrome start their periods at the same age as girls without a learning disability (age of onset 10-14 years). The majority have normal regular periods, but a significant number may have some problems. With good support and information young women with Down syndrome are able to make a successful transition into womanhood.

If the woman experiences early onset of periods (before age 10 years) or delayed periods (after age 18 years), irregular or heavy bleeding, painful periods or premenstrual tension then a medical assessment should be sought. Should a physical examination be required then counselling and education may be needed so that the woman knows what to expect. A number of visits to the doctor may be needed before a pelvic examination is undertaken. If the insertion of a speculum is not possible then sedation or external ultrasonography (a procedure where sound waves are used to produce images on a screen) may be necessary. Whether adolescent girls with Down syndrome should be seen routinely for a pelvic examination remains controversial. When prescribing medication for gynaecological reasons, doctors must consider other health problems such as epilepsy and diabetes.

Premenstrual syndrome (tension) (PMS)
Emotional and physical changes occurring one or two weeks before menstruation and vanishes either shortly before or shortly after the start of menstrual flow.

Causes: Cause is unknown, but probably related to hormonal changes associated with the normal menstrual cycle.

Symptoms and signs: Common symptoms include headaches, bloating, weight gain, breast tenderness, mood changes, fatigue, backache, lower abdominal pain and changes in behaviour.

Investigations: For several consecutive months close monitoring of the menstrual cycle and any emotional and behavioural changes should be undertaken. Similar pattern of changes should be seen over the monitoring period.

Complications: There may be an association accident proneness. PMS can lead to a deterioration of epilepsy and a misdiagnosis of mood or behaviour changes.

Treatment and prevention: Supportive therapy can be provided, including understanding, explanation, evaluation, reassurance and informational counselling. Aerobic exercise has been found in some research studies to be helpful. Some PMS symptoms may be relieved by a reduction of caffeine, sugar and sodium intake, increase of fibre and adequate rest and sleep.

Dietary intervention studies indicate that calcium supplementation (1200 mg/d) may be useful. Also vitamin E (400 IU/d) has shown some effectiveness. Antidepressants can be used to treat severe PMS. Hormonal intervention may take many forms. Hormonal contraception is commonly used, the most common forms being the combined oral contraceptive pill and the contraceptive patch. Diuretics have been used to handle water retention and non-steroidal anti-inflammatory drugs (NSAIDs; eg, ibuprofen) to treat pain. Evening primrose oil, which contains the Omega-6 EFA GLA (gamma-Linolenic acid) lacks clear scientific support.

Painful periods (dysmenorrhoea)
Common in women with Down syndrome.

Causes: These are usually related to hormonal changes and can be associated with premenstrual tension. Late onset dysmenorrhoea can be due to an underlying medical cause (eg infection, hormonal imbalance).

Symptoms and signs: There may be cramp-like pain in the lower abdomen, backache, headache, nausea, vomiting, irritability and changes in behaviour. In some women, other symptoms occur as well as pain: headaches, tiredness, feeling faint, breast tenderness, feeling sick, bloating, diarrhoea and emotional changes.

Investigations: Serious underlying causes are excluded by ultrasound examination (procedure using sound waves transmitted to body to produce pictures) and/or by laparoscopy (examination of abdomen and pelvis directly by using a flexible tube). A specialist assessment may be necessary.

Complications: These can include emotional distress or other complications which are secondary to an underlying cause.

Treatment and prevention: Mild painkillers (aspirin, naproxen), rest and using a hot-water bottle can be beneficial. Anti-inflammatory medication such as Mefenamic Acid (Ponstan) can give some relief. Supplementation with vitamin B1 or fish oils can help some women. If severe, ovulation can be stopped by use of the oral contraceptive pill. A transcutaneous electrical nerve stimulation (TENS) machine is an option for women who prefer not to use medication. These machines give out a small electrical current which seem to work by interfering with pain signals sent to the brain from the nerves.

Absence of menstrual periods (amenorrhoea)
Condition where there are no periods before the age of 16 years or where periods which previously occurred now stop.

Causes: Many causes are possible including delayed puberty, stress, pregnancy, menopause, hysterectomy, an underlying medical cause, eg hypothyroidism, adrenal gland disorder, ovary disorder, depression, drugs, anorexia and the continuous use of the oral contraceptive pill. Often however, no underlying cause is found. For some women with a learning disability antipsychotic medication may be the cause.

Symptoms and signs: Periods are absent and there may be other symptoms due to an underlying cause.

Investigations: (See painful periods above). The level of the female sex hormones in blood can be measured.

Complications: These will be secondary to the underlying cause.

Treatment: Reassurance should be given and any underlying cause treated.

Irregular periods (oligomenorrhoea)

Infrequent and unexpected periods.

Causes: Causes include: stress, the oral contraceptive pill, the menopause; medical causes such as thyroid disease, polycystic ovary syndrome, pelvic infection and the side-effects of drugs. Often no cause can be found.

Symptoms and signs: There is bleeding between periods, or whilst on the contraceptive pill.

Investigations/Complications: (see dysmenorrhoea above).

Treatment: Reassurance should be provided and the cause treated if known. The oral contraceptive pill can regulate periods.

Heavy periods (menorrhagia)

Difficult to define due to large differences between women.

Causes: This can be due to hormonal imbalance, pelvic infection, thyroid disease and stress. A cause may not be found.

Symptoms and signs: It is difficult to assess accurately, but a good indication is an increased use of tampons or sanitary pads.

Investigations: (See dysmenorrhoea above). A sample of tissue from the uterus by 'D and C' (dilation of the cervix and removal of material from the inner wall of the uterus) can help to determine cause.

Complications: The woman can develop anaemia.

Treatment: The underlying cause should be treated, if known, the combined oral contraceptive pill can reduce menorrhagia. The levonorgestrel-releasing intrauterine system (LNG-IUS) is a small plastic device that is placed in the womb and slowly releases a hormone called progestogen which leads to less womb growth and in turn less bleeding. The mini pill contains progesterone and often results in no periods. A hysterectomy will stop periods. Iron replacement can be provided for anaemia. A specialist doctor may suggest surgery if medications are not effective.

Endometriosis

Condition in which fragments of the lining of the uterus are found outside the womb.

Causes: Unknown.

Symptoms and signs: Sometimes there are none present, but causes can commonly include abnormal or heavy periods, severe abdominal pain, diarrhoea or constipation, urinary urgency, frequency, and sometimes painful voiding.

Complications: Endometriosis can cause cysts and it also increases the risk of infertility. Research has demonstrated an association between endometriosis and certain types of cancers, notably some types of ovarian cancer, non-Hodgkin's lymphoma and brain cancer.

Investigations: A gynaecological assessment is needed. Laparoscopy (examination of the inside of the abdomen with a viewing instrument) will show lesions. Use of imaging tests may identify endometriosis cysts or larger endometriosis areas. Common imaging tests used include ultrasound and magnetic resonance imaging (MRI). Normal results do not eliminate the possibility of endometriosis as endometric lesions are often too small to be seen by these tests.

Treatment: Drugs and hormonal treatments can be given to stop periods. Keyhole surgery to look into the pelvis can show lesions which can then be removed. A hysterectomy can be considered. Symptoms are often resolved once a woman reaches the menopause.

Menopause

Cluster of symptoms around time of last period due to stopping of normal function of ovaries. In females with Down syndrome the age of menopause can be 10 years earlier than for the general population. Twelve menstrual cycles have to be missed for the diagnosis to be made.

Causes: The menopause is due to natural and normal changes in sexual hormones with age.

Symptoms and signs: Some women may experience no symptoms other than irregular periods and then total cessation of periods. Other symptoms include fluid retention, palpitations, sweating, hot flushes, headaches, breast discomfort, sleep disturbance and changes in behaviour or mood.

Complications: There is increased risk of osteoporosis (bone loss) and also of hypertension.

Investigations: Usually none is required but thyroid or psychological conditions can be excluded if necessary. A blood test for follicle stimulating hormone (FSH) can be done.

Treatment: Reassurance and explanation can help and hormone replacement therapy (HRT), drugs to protect bones or antidepressants may be given.

Candida Infection (Candidiasis; Thrush)

Causes: Yeast infection called Candida albicans. Normally found on and in the body. Everyone carries this organism on their skin, in their mouth, in their gastrointestinal tract, and women in their vagina. Risk factors for an infection include poor hygiene, the use of antibiotics and obesity.

Symptoms and signs: There may be irritation and redness of the vulvae, discharge, odour, itching, bleeding, pain on urination and changes in behaviour or mood.

Complications: The infection can spread to others.

Investigations: A sample of the vaginal discharge is sent to the lab for examination under the microscope and to grow candida.

Treatment and prevention: Reassurance and explanation should be provided and antifungal medication creams (eg Mycostatin), vaginal suppositories (eg Monistat), mild topical steroid, oral medication can be prescribed. Prevention is important and includes simple advice, eg, wearing loose cotton underwear, avoiding tights and tight underwear, eating live yogurt, cutting down on sugar, changing the contraceptive pill prescribed and reducing the intake of antibiotics for viral infections, eg a cold or the flu.

Sexual health issues for men

Hypospadias

Opening of the urethra usually on the underside of the penis. The penis may also curve downwards. Opening on top of penis is rare and known as epispadias.

Causes: The condition is present at birth.

Symptoms and signs: Problems can occur on passing urine and achieving an erection may be difficult.

Investigations/Complications: There are usually none but approximately 10% of boys with hypospadias have at least one undescended testis, and a similar number have an inguinal hernia. If the hypospadias is severe (scrotal or perineal) urinary tract infections, renal stone formation can occur.

Treatment: If the condition is causing concern a surgical correction procedure can take place (usually however this is done as an infant).

Phimosis

A condition where the foreskin of the penis is tight and there is difficulty in drawing it back over the head of the penis. Normally diagnosed in infants.

Causes: The condition can be present at birth. In adults it can be due to skin disease, inflammation of the penis or scarring of the foreskin due to previous forced withdrawal.

Symptoms and signs: There is difficulty in passing urine, ballooning out of foreskin on urination, difficulty in achieving a full erection.

Investigations: None are usually required.

Complications: Occasionally an infection or urinary retention can occur.

Treatment: The problem can improve over time without medical intervention. Gently withdrawing the foreskin when in the bath (do not force) can be helpful for minor conditions. Application of topical steroid cream, such as betamethasone, for 4–6 weeks to the narrow part of the foreskin is relatively simple and is known to be effective. Severe cases may require a circumcision (removal of a part of the foreskin of the penis).

Undescended testis

Failure of the testis to be present in the scrotum usually affects one testis only but can affect both. Testes usually descend by seven months of age.

Causes: The condition is present at birth. Risk factors include low birth weight, maternal diabetes, and premature birth.

Symptoms and signs: Usually this causes no pain or any symptoms. Palpable undescended testicles are located just above the scrotum.

Investigations: None are usually required.

Complications: Impaired sperm production and an increased risk of testicular cancer have been reported. Self-esteem issues may be of concern to teenagers with Down syndrome.

Treatment: Surgical intervention can be considered to lower the testis into the scrotum but should be weighed up against the risk of surgery and the benefits of the procedure.

Candida Infection (Candidiasis; Thrush)

Causes: (See sexual health for women above). Less common in men than women.

Symptoms and signs: In men it usually affects the head of the penis causing inflammation, a smelly lumpy discharge, pain while passing urine and changes in behaviour or mood.

Complications: The infection can spread to others and to internal organs.

Investigations: A sample of the discharge is examined under the microscope and cultured to grow candida.

Treatment and prevention: Reassurance and explanation should be provided and antifungal medication prescribed such as fluconazole (Diflucan). Prevention is cleaning the penis regularly, avoid perfumed shower gels or soaps on the penis, as they can cause irritation. Make sure penis is dried properly after washing. Loose-fitting cotton underwear can help prevent moisture building up under the foreskin, which lowers the risk of the infection.

Sexual health promotion

It is important that people with a learning disability are able to benefit from the same health education and prevention measures as everyone else. Regular check-ups are an essential part of maintaining good sexual health in order that treatment can be carried out if necessary. Coupled with education into the reasons for such check-ups, the person with a learning disability should be helped to understand the risks to health that are posed by such agents as smoking and unprotected sex.

For women, breast checks in the form of breast examination once a month are important as the first step in detecting problems. Some women with Down syndrome will be able to carry out the check-ups by themselves, while others may need help from family members or paid staff and yearly examinations by a doctor. All women with Down syndrome should also be enabled to participate in breast screening programmes at the same intervals as the general population. A number of accessible guides for women on how to do a regular breast examination are available. For more information see Appendix D.

Cervical smear tests likewise aim to detect changes that may become cancerous so that early treatment may be carried out. Preparation is necessary to ensure that the woman understands what is involved in a pelvic examination. Again information on accessible materials is available in Appendix D.

As with breast checks by women, some men will be able to examine their own testicles while others will need to be examined by a doctor or a specialist nurse. Men with Down syndrome are reported to have an increased risk of testicular cancer. Therefore information and support to undertake regular examination is important. Information on accessible materials is available in Appendix D.

Contraception

Women with Down syndrome should receive information and advice about the range of contraceptive options that are available to them in a way that best suits their communication needs.

For many women the oral contraceptive pill remains the first choice. Benefits of the pill include reduced dysmenorrhoea (period pain), reduced infection and reduced risk of ovarian cancer. However, side-effects such as nausea, headache, thrombosis and hypertension can occur and a history of seizures, liver disease, or cardiovascular disease may prevent the use of the pill. Important interactions with other drugs such as anti-convulsants (group of drugs used to treat epilepsy, for example carbamazepine, sodium valproate, phenytoin) can also occur.

Intrauterine devices are of limited use in people with a learning disability. Increased dysmenorrhoea and infections can be quite serious in people with reduced awareness of possible symptoms. Insertion and regular checkups may be upsetting for some women with a learning disability.

Depo-Provera, a long-acting form of the contraceptive pill injected into the muscle, is available. It is an injection of the hormone progestogen given once every three months. It is reliable and there are no proven side-effects apart from those similar to the oral contraceptive pill (above). It can be used as an alternative for women for whom an oestrogen containing pill is contraindicated.

Barrier methods (condoms, diaphragms) can be of value but require consistent attention to practice and a degree of self discipline that may be difficult for some people with a learning disability. Training and practice for both partners may be necessary.

There is a considerable amount of information for people with learning disabilities on contraception and other sexual health issues and organisations across the UK which provide specialist services. Some of these are included in the appendices to this book and you will find additional information about local and national services on the internet.

Sterilisation

Family members and paid staff are sometimes concerned about a woman with Down syndrome becoming pregnant or a man with Down Syndrome fathering a child and sometimes people ask about sterilisation. Professional medical and advocacy support for the person and their family may be required if the risks of unwanted pregnancy are high. Alternatives should be fully explored. If a person with Down syndrome understands all aspects of the procedure for sterilisation (tubal ligation for women, vasectomy for men) and can give informed consent the procedure may be carried out. Informed consent means that they must understand that the procedure involves an operation with the result that they will never be able to have children. If informed consent for this particular decision is not possible then, in the UK, legal action through the Court has to be undertaken in line with the legislation on mental capacity for the country the person lives in.

Sexually transmitted diseases

While chlamydia, gonorrhoea and syphilis are easily treatable if the symptoms are recognised, symptoms of some other sexually transmitted diseases are not so obvious. A person infected with HIV virus can, at the moment, only receive treatment that slows down the progress of the disease.

It is therefore vitally important that people with a learning disability are helped to understand the means and risk of catching a sexually transmitted disease and the ways in which such risks may be avoided or reduced such as the use of condoms, maintaining a monogamous relationship, or not having sexual intercourse.

Sexual abuse

Women and men with Down syndrome are reported to be at greater risk of suffering sexual violence or abuse, but may often be unable to tell others about what has happened due to difficulties in communication, understanding what has taken place, mental trauma and fear of reprisal. Changes in behaviour may be the first sign to suggest sexual violence or abuse has occurred. Such changes may include:

- changes in emotional behaviour, eg becoming more irritable and moody
- depression
- social isolation
- self-harm
- increase in self-talking

- negative thoughts and comments
- loss of skills and need for more comfort and support
- refusal to take part in day-to-day activities
- contact with the police for minor offences

If sexual abuse is suspected then support workers working for an organisation will need to follow the safeguarding and adult protection policies and procedures of their organisation. This is important as a medical assessment is necessary as soon as possible to screen for injuries, identify medical evidence, prosecute the offender, reassure the victim and families and to initiate safeguarding and police involvement. Accident and emergency departments are best suited to undertake the medical assessment.

People who are abused will require a considerable amount of support and counselling to come to terms with their trauma and to regain their self-esteem. Professionals, including the police, are now trained in providing the necessary support.

Chapter 10

Urinary system

Several problems of the urinary system can occur in adults with Down syndrome. Many of these will be present from birth. These include a reduced weight and size of the kidneys, dilation and obstruction of the kidney vessels and simple kidney cysts. The presence of structural abnormalities at any site of the urinary system (Figure 9) will increase susceptibility to impaired kidney function and increase the risk of infections.

Figure 9: **Structures of the urinary system**

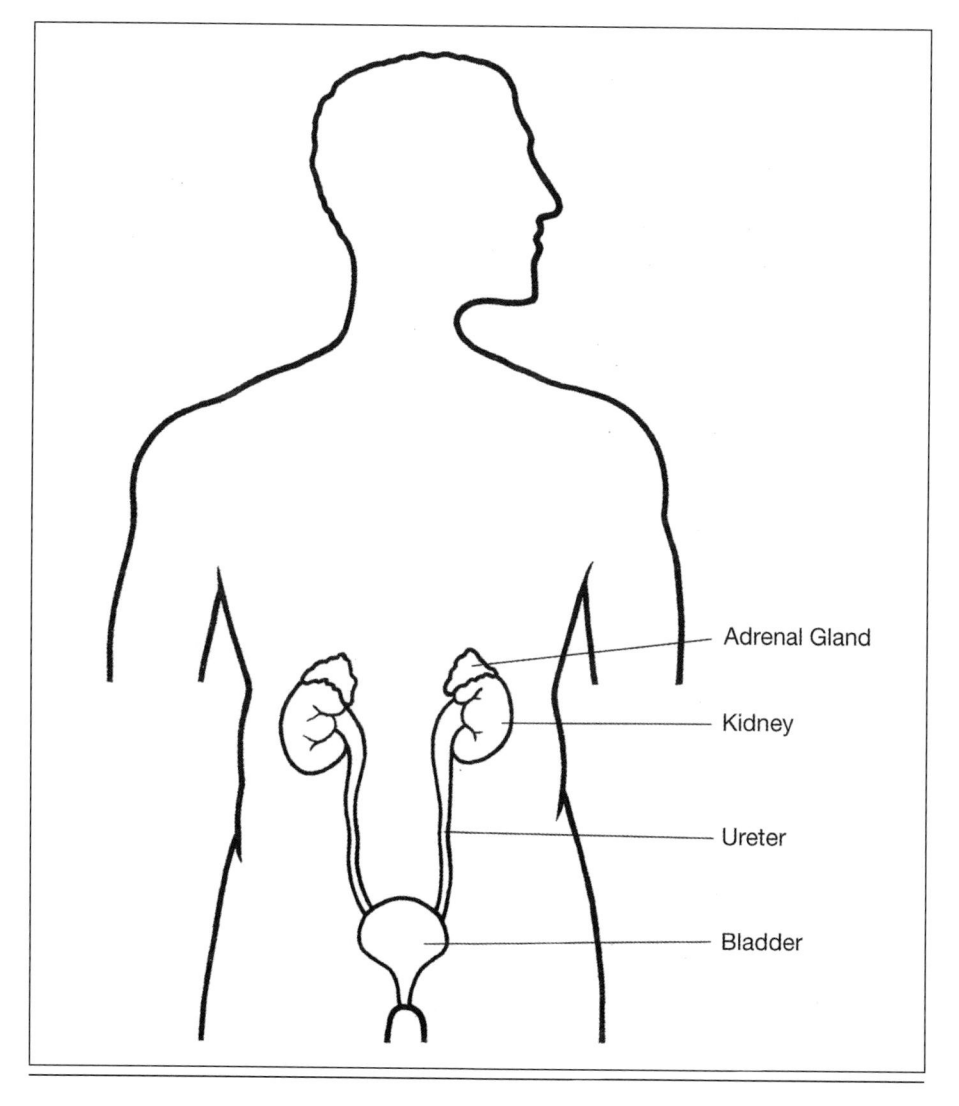

Urinary tract infection
Kidney, urinary tract and bladder infections are common in adults with Down syndrome.

Causes: The majority of infections have no identifiable cause, and single infections do not cause any significant damage. When the cause is known it is usually due to bacteria from the person's own bowel area. Factors include poor personal hygiene, chemicals in bath water, wearing of continence pads or sanitary towels and use of a urinary catheter. Less common, but more important causes include abnormalities present at birth, kidney stones and a bladder obstruction. Recurrent infections can occur in persons who 'hold-on' to their urine.

Symptoms and signs: Usually there is an increased frequency of passing urine by day and night, pain on passing urine, abdominal pain and tenderness, blood in urine, urge to pass urine and smelly urine. These symptoms suggest a lower tract infection or 'cystitis', but an infection of the kidneys can cause loin pain and tenderness usually with a fever. Occasionally infections can present with no symptoms. Behavioural and/or emotional changes can be caused by a urinary tract infection.

Complications: The important complications include spread of the infection into the blood stream (septicaemia), shock or a scarring anywhere along the urinary system.

Investigations: These involve trying to detect the type of infection and whether any damage has been caused. Tests include an analysis of a mid-stream specimen of urine for bacteria, cystoscopy (tube passed into the bladder), ultrasound scanning (procedure where sound waves are used to produce pictures) and an abdominal x-ray examination.

Treatment: A high fluid intake and regular emptying of the bladder can help to flush out any bacteria. A potassium citrate mixture and/or antibiotics (eg amoxicillin, trimethoprim) may be prescribed. Someone who is acutely ill may require admission to hospital. For individuals with recurrent infections an investigation should be made for a cause, eg stones, birth abnormalities in the structure of the urinary system.

Urinary tract obstruction

This can occur anywhere between the kidney and urethral outlet, leading to dilation of the tract above the obstruction and impaired kidney function.

Causes: These include: those inside the tract, eg stones, blood clot, in rare cases a tumour; a problem within the wall of the tract, eg muscle dysfunction, stricture, pin-hole outlet or causes outside the tract, eg an enlarged prostate.

Symptoms and signs: There may be loin pain, inability to urinate or reduced urine output, infection, difficulty in passing urine, a need to pass urine often and incontinence. The condition can cause severe distress and behavioural and emotional changes.

Investigations: Blood tests are used especially for urea and creatinine levels (measures of kidney function). The site and cause of the obstruction can be detected by ultrasonography (procedure using sound waves to produce pictures), by x-ray examination of the urinary system or cystoscopy (small tube with camera passed through urethra into bladder).

Complications: If untreated the condition can lead to kidney failure (below).

Treatment: Any obstruction needs to be relieved and any underlying cause treated. This may require surgical intervention. Urine flow can be improved with medication if enlarged prostate is cause. Any associated infection should be treated.

Kidney failure

An inability of the kidneys to excrete bodily waste products. The onset can be sudden (acute) or gradual (chronic).

Causes: a) Acute kidney failure may be due to a range of causes which include pre-kidney problems (eg hypotension, blood infection), kidney problems (eg infection) and post-kidney problems (eg urinary tract obstruction). b) The common causes of chronic kidney failure include kidney inflammation, infection, diabetes, hypertension, long-standing urinary tract obstruction and medications.

Symptoms and signs: These include malaise, anorexia, decreased or increased urine output, nausea and vomiting, water retention, breathlessness, anaemia, and hypertension. Behavioural and/or emotional changes can occur.

Investigations: Severity and any deterioration in kidney function should be monitored. Regular examination of the urine and blood biochemistry (particularly for urea and creatinine-measures of kidney function) is necessary. Ultrasound (sound waves transmitted to body and reflected back to produce images), x-ray/MRI examination or a small sample of kidney tissue (kidney biopsy) may be undertaken. Regular blood pressure measurements are necessary to detect hypertension.

Complications: If kidney failure is not treated an imbalance of the body's blood chemistry will result and is life threatening.

Treatment: Acute kidney failure is a medical emergency and requires immediate hospital management, eg replace lost fluid, surgically remove obstruction. In chronic kidney failure underlying causes should be treated. Blood pressure control, dietary advice, use of diuretics and steroids are important to good management. If there is severe kidney failure, haemodialysis (removal of toxins from the blood by means of being attached to a specially designed machine) or a kidney transplant should be considered.

Prostate enlargement
The prostate gland is a gland found in men around the urinary tract which produces the fluid that carries sperm. A normal enlargement occurs in men with age, termed 'benign prostatic hyperplasia (BPH)' or 'benign prostatic hypertrophy'.

Causes: It is usually related to hormonal changes with age, but occasionally can be due to cancer.

Symptoms and signs: Frequent urination, waking at night to go to the toilet, delay in initiating urination, reduced force, and dribbling are frequent symptoms. There may be dribbling at the end of urinating, pain with urination or bloody urine (these may indicate infection).

Investigations: A manual examination of the prostate via the rectum can often detect an enlarged gland. An x-ray examination, cystourethroscopy (passing of flexible tube through urethra to visualise the lower urinary system) and/or scans can be performed to confirm any enlargement, the reason for enlargement and any effects due to the swelling. Urine examination and blood tests (urea and creatinine levels) should be undertaken to assess kidney function. A blood test can be done to detect a marker for prostate cancer; if this is suspected biopsies may be taken.

Complications: An obstruction of the bladder outflow can lead to bladder distension. The condition can occasionally lead to kidney failure (above).

Treatment: If the enlargement is mild it can be treated with simple measures such as: encouraging the person to urinate when he first gets the urge, to go to the bathroom when he has the chance, to avoid alcohol and caffeine, not to drink a lot of fluid all at once, to avoid cold and sinus medications that contain decongestants or antihistamines, to keep warm and exercise regularly.
Cold weather and lack of physical activity may worsen symptoms. Learning and performing pelvic strengthening exercises and reducing stress can help. Nervousness and tension can lead to more frequent urination. Drugs such as Alpha 1-blockers (eg doxazosin, prazosin) can relax the muscles of the bladder neck and prostate. This allows easier urination. Finasteride and dutasteride lower levels of hormones produced by the prostate reduce the size of the prostate gland, increase urine flow rate. Antibiotics may be prescribed to treat chronic prostatitis (inflammation of the prostate), which may accompany prostatic enlargement. A significant enlarged prostate will require surgery intervention (transurethral resection). If cancer is present surgical removal of the prostate (prostatectomy) and radiotherapy is required.

Chapter 11

Nervous system

The nervous system consists of the brain, the spinal cord and numerous smaller nerves which are widespread over the body. The nervous system interacts with virtually all other systems in the body and therefore has a significant role to play in the health status of a person. Clear information from the person with Down syndrome and from their family members and support staff is most important in understanding the potential cause of any problem. Medical attention should always be sought for any condition giving cause for concern.

Headache

Produced by stimulation of pain-sensitive structures within the skull or tissue around the skull. Often under-reported by adults with Down syndrome; this could be because they experience them less, have difficulty identifying a headache and subsequently seeking help, or they may have a higher threshold for pain.

Causes: A single episode is common, and can vary from a minor complaint to a serious acute emergency. Attention needs to be paid to the site, the suddenness of onset, and to any associated fever or rash. A severe single episode of a headache may be due to a number of causes such as toothache or following head trauma. Less obvious, but more serious causes can be due to life threatening conditions such as a stroke, brain haemorrhage or meningitis.

Recurrent headaches may be due to recurrent ear infections (Chapter 5), impaired visual acuity (sharpness of vision), sinusitis, atlanto-axial instability (AAI; Chapter 12), glaucoma (Chapter 4), side-effects of medication, migraine or tension.

Symptoms and signs: Tension headaches and headaches due to eyestrain usually present as 'a tight band' around the head, pressure behind the eyes, throbbing or as a bursting sensation. Migraine attacks can present with features prior to the headache of visual symptoms, speech difficulties, nausea, vomiting or irritability. Symptoms of an underlying cause may be present, eg tender cheekbones in sinusitis.

Investigations: Investigations are often not necessary but this depends on the cause. They can include blood tests, skull and upper neck x-ray (when a head injury has occurred or is suspected), CT or MRI brain scan and a lumbar puncture (procedure to take fluid from around the spine from the lower back).

Complications: Most headaches are self-limiting. Complications can follow meningitis or a brain haemorrhage.

Treatment and prevention: These depend on the type of headache. Tension headaches can benefit from reassurance, avoiding the cause, analgesia, physical treatment (massage, relaxation), increased fluid intake, sleep and, if required, from a course of antidepressants (drugs used to treat depression). Migraine headaches can benefit from reassurance, avoiding dietary triggering foods, paracetamol and prophylactic medication to prevent migraine.

Following serious head trauma, or if a headache is associated with vomiting, disturbed consciousness or visual loss an urgent medical assessment is recommended.

Unconsciousness
Altered state of alertness.

Causes: **Concussion** is a brief loss of consciousness due to a head injury, eg owing to a fall, traffic accident. Usually there is no associated damage, but the person should be observed closely and the doctor informed. **Fainting** is a temporary loss of consciousness due to poor oxygen supply to the brain. This can be due to pain, stress, shock, fear, prolonged coughing or straining, low blood pressure, medication, heart disease, hypothyroidism or diabetes (Chapter 14). **Coma** is a loss of consciousness with a lack of response to stimuli, eg pinching or shouting. A coma is usually due to a more serious condition including severe head injury, seizures, build up of poisons (eg drugs, liver or kidney failure), diabetes, brain infection or meningitis. After a **seizure**, loss of consciousness is common and can last from a few minutes to several hours.

Investigations: Severity and cause need to be determined. Tests can include blood and urine analysis for diabetes, hormones and major organ function. More detailed tests include electroencephalography (EEG, investigation of the brain function by measurement of electrical brain activity), a brain CT or MRI scan and a lumbar puncture (procedure to take fluid from around the spine from the lower back).

Complications: These depend on the cause, but if medical treatment is not obtained unconsciousness can prove to be fatal.

Treatment: **Concussion**: Resting for 24 hours under supervision is usually adequate. If there is disturbed breathing, vomiting, problems with vision then see a doctor for further assessment. **Fainting**: The person should sit down and lean forward, head down between knees or alternatively lie down and raise their legs. If they are unconscious for several minutes seek medical help. Seizure: (see below). After the immediate management a further detailed medical assessment will be required. Information regarding diabetic status, epilepsy, medication, and trauma is essential. **Coma:** Check breathing and that the airway is clear. If the person is not breathing start resuscitation procedures, if you have been trained to carry these out. Seek urgent medical assistance. If the person is breathing normally place them into the 'recovery position' as follows:

- lay the person on their back, turn their head onto their left side
- put their left arm by their side and slide it under their buttock
- lay their right arm across chest and cross their right leg over left leg
- from the left side, lean over and grasp clothes at hip and pull the person over onto their left side
- bend the person's right arm and right leg to give support, free left arm and keep head tilted back and airway clear.
- seek medical help, do not leave the person alone; no food or drink should be given.

Epilepsy (seizures)
A neurological condition characterised by a convulsive attack and change in consciousness.

Causes: Changes in the electrical discharge in the brain can lead to an altered level of consciousness and abnormal movements (a seizure).

Single seizure: Seizures can be triggered by a trauma, fever, infections, drugs (eg anti-dementia drugs, antidepressants), physical illness, stroke or heart disease.

Recurrent seizures: Overall these are probably more common in people with Down syndrome than in the general population. There appear to be three age peaks, in infants, young adults and the older population. For the older population tonic-clonic and myoclonic seizures are common (often associated with Alzheimer's disease – Chapter 15). A cause often is not identified and probably relates to the different structure, electrical wiring and chemical makeup in adults with Down syndrome as compared to the general population.

Seizure types:

- **Generalised** (whole of brain affected and consciousness lost).
- **Tonic-clonic:** The person loses consciousness, stiffens, falls and limbs jerk.
- **Myoclonic:** There are uncontrollable jerks.
- **Atonic:** This involves a loss of muscle tone and the person falls down.
- **Absences:** The person is temporally unresponsive, staring. No falling occurs but there may be associated jerking of an arm. The seizure cannot be interrupted by talking or touching and usually last 10 seconds, but several seizures can occur each day.
- **Partial seizures** (only a limited part of the brain is affected. Localised unusual symptoms can be experienced, eg tingling, flashing lights can occur).
  - Simple partial seizure – symptoms of a partial seizure, but the person remains conscious.
  - Complex partial seizure – symptoms of a partial seizure, but there is a loss of awareness.
- **Secondary generalised seizures.** A partial seizure (above) spreads to involve the whole of the brain and there are features also of a generalised seizure.

Investigations: A detailed history of the seizure is important. Videotaping episodes can be extremely useful. Other tests include an electrogram (EEG - recording of the electrical brain pattern), CT or MRI brain scan, blood screen and blood anticonvulsant drug levels.

Complications: Injury, choking, behaviour and emotional changes are common. Status epilepticus (repeated seizures without full recovery between each) is a serious complication. Epilepsy can lead to death if severe complications occur or if seizures are severe or prolonged.

Treatment and prevention: First aid is required, this varies depending on type of seizure. It may include: cushioning the person's head (with hands if nothing else is available). They should not be physically restrained or moved during a seizure, nothing should be put into the mouth and tight clothing should be loosened. When the attack has finished the person should be placed on their side in the recovery position (for details see above) and should not be left alone until fully recovered. For prolonged seizures an ambulance or medical help should be called. Rectal diazepam or oral midazolam (syringed into the mouth) can be given to stop the immediate seizures. Long-term treatment will involve taking anticonvulsant drugs (group of drugs used to treat epilepsy, eg diazepam, carbamazepine, sodium valproate) either to stop a seizure or to try to prevent future seizures. For more information go to www.epilepsysociety.org.uk/first-aid-all-seizure-types.

Change in diet or psychological support can also be of benefit. For extreme cases where medication has failed and seizures continue to be severe, brain surgery or a procedure called vagus nerve stimulation can be proposed. Vagus nerve stimulation therapy involves a stimulator (called a pulse generator) placed in the chest wall with a wire connected to the left vagus nerve in the neck (a nerve from the brain). The pulse generator sends regular electrical stimulation to the nerve and reduces seizures. The regular recording of seizure frequency is important.

An identification card and education for family members and support workers on how to deal with seizures can aid management. Regular medical reviews of drug therapy including routine blood tests are necessary to prevent toxicity, reduce side-effects and stop drug interactions. Extra supervision and care is necessary when a person with seizures undertakes swimming or activities where becoming unconscious could cause serious harm. Special care should be taken if a woman with Down syndrome is considering having a child as some anti-epileptics can be harmful to the baby. Barrier methods of contraception should be considered as some anti-epileptics reduce the effectiveness of the oral contraceptive pill.

Myoclonus
Sudden jerking of a muscle or group of muscles.

Causes: Can occur in healthy people, but seen commonly in adults with Down syndrome as part of a seizure or as part of Alzheimer's disease (Chapter 15).

Symptoms and signs: 'Jumps' or sudden involuntary jerking of usually an arm or a leg occur. Night-time jerks are common and do not suggest any serious problem.

Investigations: An underlying medical cause should be excluded, in particular epilepsy or Alzheimer's disease. An EEG can help to decide if the 'jumps' are seizures.

Complications: Often there are none, but occasionally a generalised convulsion can be triggered (see epilepsy above).

Treatment and prevention: Reassurance may be all that is necessary. Anticonvulsant medication will be prescribed including clonazepam, sodium valproate, piracetam, and primidone. Hormonal therapy also may improve responses to anti-myoclonic drugs in some people.

Stroke

Damage to the brain due to disruption in the blood supply to the brain.

Causes: Blood vessels supplying oxygen to the brain are blocked and lead to a part of the brain dying (infarction) or bleeding from the blood vessels into the brain resulting in damage to brain tissue. Unlike in the general population, atheroma (hardening of arteries) is uncommon in adults with Down syndrome. Blood clots breaking away from a heart which has birth defects and travelling up to the brain are often the cause of a stroke. Mini strokes called 'transient ischemic attacks' or TIAs lead to a short duration of symptoms and usually/often full recovery is seen.

Symptoms and signs: These depend on which part of the brain is affected, but commonly include weakness down one side of the body, speech impairment, confusion, visual problems.

Investigations: An underlying medical cause should be excluded and the severity of damage assessed. CT or MRI brain scans can show-up damage to the brain.

Complications: Strokes are a major cause of death and physical disability.

Treatment and prevention: Rapid assessment in hospital is vital if a stroke is suspected. Early treatment to try and break up a clot will improve the outcome. On admission a patient with signs of a stroke should have an urgent CT scan. If no bleed is seen and it is less than three hours since the symptoms started, it is likely the diagnosis is a clot causing a stroke and the patient can be 'thrombolysed' (a medication given into the veins which breaks up the clot). A bleed causing the stroke may require neurosurgical input. Once stabilisation has occurred rehabilitation is important to improve any motor, speech, and visual disabilities. Physiotherapy, speech and language therapy and occupational therapy can help a person cope better with their impairments. There is an increased risk of a further stroke, so preventative medications should be given (statins).

Restless legs syndrome
Neurological disorder with irresistible urge to move one's body to stop uncomfortable sensations.

Causes: Often no cause is identified, but the condition does increase with age.

Symptoms and signs: There is a repeated desire to move the legs, but it can affect the arms and torso and is worse at rest and at night.

Investigations: Vitamin deficiencies should be ruled out, eg iron deficiency.

Complications: None, but the condition can have a fluctuating course for many years.

Treatment and prevention: Simple measures such as regular exercise, leg massage, keeping legs warm can help. Medication can be prescribed (ropinirole).

Chapter 12

Skeleton, joints and dental care

Skeletal and joint problems are common in adults with Down syndrome because of the differences in bone and tissue structure and because of their reduced muscle tone. The majority of problems can be attributed to the 'looseness' of ligaments secondary to changes in collagen (the building block of ligaments and muscles).

Skeleton and joints

Dislocation of joints

This is the displacement of two bones in a joint. Commonly dislocated joints are the knee, hip, elbow, patella, spine and thumb.

Causes: Dislocation is due to 'loose' joints because of increased elasticity of ligaments and reduced muscle tone.

Symptoms and signs: These include pain, weakness and loss of movement, misshapen joints, the person holding the limb in an odd position, swelling, inability to weight bear, abnormal walking stance, incontinence of urine and/or bowels, distress and disturbed behaviour.

Investigations: An x-ray or CT/MRI scan of the joint will show any abnormality present.

Complications: Nerve damage and paralysis or damage to the blood supply is uncommon, but can occur. Repeated dislocations can lead to degeneration of the joint.

Treatment and prevention: Minor dislocations may manipulate back by themselves. For others a splint may be needed to stop further movement and secondary damage, until manipulated back by a doctor. There should be no eating or drinking before treatment as a general anaesthesia may be given. The joint is usually manipulated back into position by a trained professional. This can be a very painful process and is therefore typically done either in the emergency department under sedation or in an operating room. For joints with repeated dislocations surgical intervention may be necessary to stabilise the joint. Improved muscle mass with physiotherapy can increase stability of joints. Care should be taken when undertaking physical activities to prevent recurrence of the dislocation.

Painful joints

Causes: A long history would suggest arthritis (see osteoarthritis, rheumatoid arthritis below), but a short sudden onset may suggest dislocation (see above) trauma (including a fracture), sprain, tendinitis, gout, septic arthritis. Pain in the arm can be due to a neck problem or a painful knee due to a hip problem.

Symptoms and signs: These include painful joints, stiffness, swelling, warmth, redness, tenderness, loss of function, behaviour and emotional changes.

Investigations: Blood tests are taken for evidence of inflammation, the presence of joint antibodies (proteins produced by the body against parts of the joint) and uric acid levels to rule out gout. An x-ray examination or CT/MRI scan of the joint, joint aspiration (small amount of fluid in joint removed by insertion of needle) may be necessary. The doctor may also undertake an arthroscopic examination. This is where a small, flexible tube is inserted into the joint through a very small skin incision to examine the interior regions.

Complications: Immobility and chronic problems can occur, if there is an underlying cause.

Treatment: The main treatment involves rest, weight loss, use of painkillers and non-steroidal anti-inflammatory drugs, eg ibuprofen (with caution), steroid-based drugs, physical therapy (heat, hydrotherapy), and physiotherapy to strengthen the muscles around the joint. Occasionally surgery (joint replacement) is necessary if problems persist.

Atlanto-occipital instability (AOI) and atlanto-axial instability (AAI)

Joints at the top of the spine and at the base of the skull allow normal nodding and shaking movements of the head (Figure 10). In individuals with Down syndrome these joints can be more lax and weaker than other joints, leading to damage to nearby nerves. Atlanto-axial instability (AAI) is more common than AOI.

Cause: Laxity of ligaments and joints.

Symptoms and signs: Usually there are none, but it can result in spinal nerves being trapped. Symptoms of spinal cord involvement are weakness in arms and/or legs, problems in walking, local neck pain and discomfort, neck stiffness, head tilt, urinary incontinence, and brisk tendon reflexes especially of the ankles, mis-diagnosis of dementia. Symptoms can occur following injury and can be quite sudden.

Investigations: X-ray or scan of the upper spine.

Complications: Dislocation of the AOI or AAI joints can lead to serious spinal cord damage with resultant permanent paralysis and can be life threatening.

Treatment and prevention: If AOI or AAI is present, then the person, together with their doctor, needs to consider exclusion from more risky sporting activities, eg gymnastics, diving, butterfly stroke in swimming, football, trampolining. Caution is required with over extension of the neck (eg when having a general anaesthetic). Head rests are useful when travelling to prevent whiplash injuries. Surgical intervention may be necessary to stabilise the joints if AAI or AOI is present and leading to nerve damage. This involves fusion with bone grafts or metal wire for the affected joints. If symptoms are chronic then surgical benefit may be limited. Screening for AOI and AAI by routine cervical x-rays is no longer recommended and is unlikely to be helpful in deciding which individuals may be at risk of nerve involvement. Medical opinion should be sought if any symptoms suggestive of cervical spine problems occur.

Figure 10: **Upper spine**

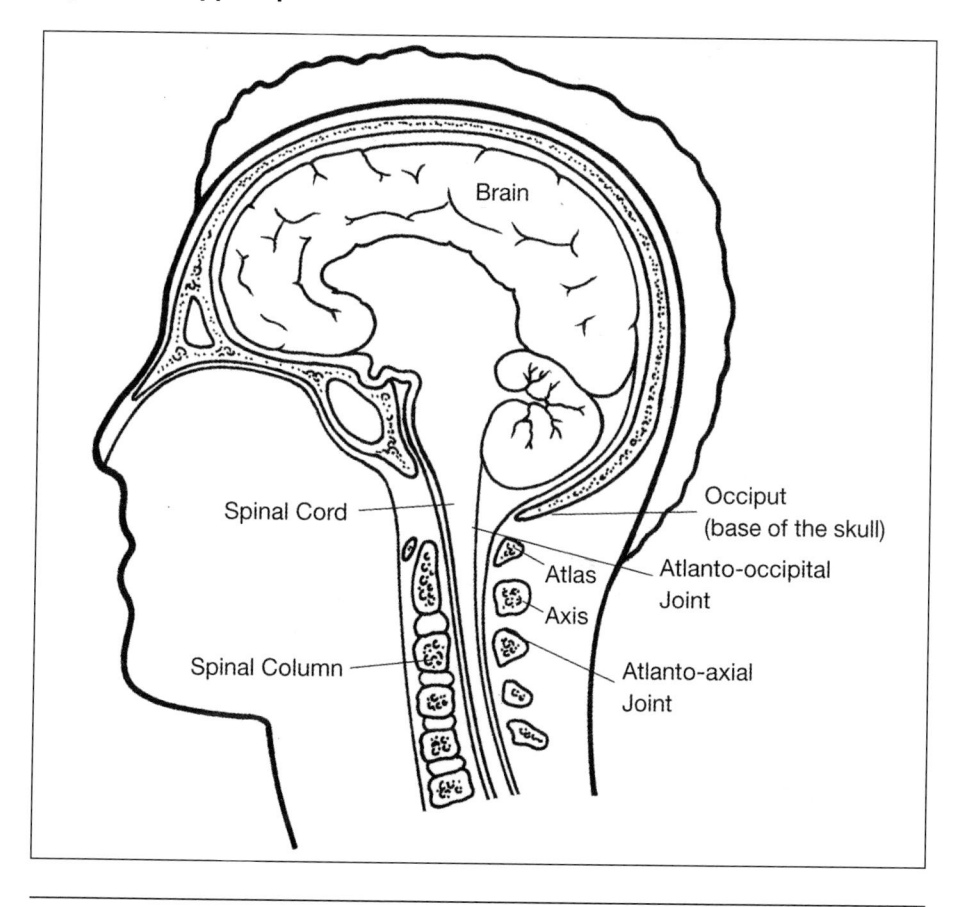

Feet problems
These include flat feet, dry feet, fissures, split nails, callosities, bunions, infection of toe-nails, wide-based walking stance and external rotation of foot.

Causes: Minor deformities are extremely common in people with Down syndrome due to looseness of ligaments, obesity and ill-fitting shoes.

Symptoms and signs: These commonly include abnormal appearance, pain in the foot, abnormal walking posture and ingrowing toe-nails.

Treatment and prevention: An assessment by a foot specialist (podiatrist) may be necessary depending on the cause, but foot exercises (eg walking on tip-toes), shoe pads or inserts or specifically designed shoes can prevent some problems. Surgical correction of deformities is occasionally required. Medication can be given for infections or to reduce any joint inflammation. Psychological intervention may be necessary to enable the person to have their toe-nails cut if they are resistant to being supported to do this.

Scoliosis
Side to side curvature of the spine, usually in the middle of the back.

Causes: The condition is present at birth; there is laxity of ligaments and poor posture.

Symptoms: These include spinal deformity, odd postures, abnormal walking.

Investigations: A spinal x-ray will show the deformity.

Complications: If minor change is present then usually there are no associated problems. If the scoliosis is severe it can lead to breathing problems, heart problems, chest discomfort and problems with balance and walking.

Treatment: If the scoliosis is mild, regular monitoring may be all that is required. Physiotherapy with targeted exercises to improve posture and muscle strength is the main treatment for most people. If the scoliosis is severe, the person may need surgical intervention with spinal fusion of the vertebrae to straighten the spine.

Osteoarthritis
'Wear and tear' inflammation and degeneration of joints; affects mainly the large joints and cervical spine.

Causes: Osteoarthritis is associated with increasing age, laxity of joints and increased dislocations, obesity and immobility.

Symptoms: (See painful joints above).

Investigations: These include x-ray or CT/MRI scan of joint, blood tests for evidence of joint inflammation and arthroscopic examination.

Complications: Osteoarthritis can lead to degeneration of the joint; nerves can become trapped.

Treatment: (See painful joints above). Additional treatments may include injections of corticosteroids into the joint, injection of hyaluronic acid, chiropractic manipulation and acupuncture.

Osteoporosis
Thinning of bones.

Causes: The condition is associated with increasing age, decrease in oestrogen after the menopause in women, poor intake of calcium and vitamin D, immobility, steroid therapy, drugs such as anti-convulsants and lithium.

Symptoms: There is often none but there may be changes in how the person walks.

Investigations: Bone density and degree of thinning of the bones can be assessed using a special x-ray test known as DEXA (dual-energy x-ray absorptiometry).

Complications: Fractures are a major concern.

Treatment and prevention: Regular exercise can improve bone density. Good intake of calcium and vitamin D (eg in fish, milk, cheese, green vegetables, fruits) is recommended. Regular exposure to sunlight can help vitamin D absorption. For women who have reached the menopause, oestrogen replacement therapy (HRT) can maintain bone strength. Drugs (such as calcitonin) can improve bone density.

Rheumatoid arthritis

An inflammation of several and usually symmetrical joints.

Causes: This is a possible autoimmune condition where the body's own defence mechanism attacks its own joints.

Symptoms and signs: These include a gradual onset of joint pain (usually hands or feet), morning stiffness, tenderness, swelling, reduced function and deformity. Joints on both sides of the body are affected at the same time.

Investigations: Elevated measures of joint inflammation in blood and evidence of abnormal defence response are investigated. There is also a test for a specific marker for rheumatoid arthritis, called 'rheumatoid factor'. An x-ray of the joints can show damage caused.

Complications: These are uncommon, but loss of function of joints, nerve compression (eg cervical spine involvement) or an inflammation of some other body organ can occur.

Treatment: (See painful joints above).

Teeth

Teeth are important in the preparation of food for swallowing and digestion, in the production of speech and also in the appearance of the individual. The latter point is important since appearance has a great deal to do with socialisation and social inclusion. Due to structural changes in the oral cavity, dry mouth (with more viscous saliva), delayed tooth eruption and missing permanent teeth, adults with Down syndrome are prone to experience more dental problems than the rest of the population. Good oral cleanliness is essential and regular assessments by a dentist are important to prevent serious health problems because of the heart conditions commonly associated with Down syndrome.

Developing and maintaining the habit of effective teeth brushing is important to ensure that dental problems are minimised. Annual checkups should take place, if necessary with a dentist who has experience in looking after people with a learning disability.

Toothache

Causes: Common conditions include tooth decay, eruption of wisdom teeth, mouth ulcers, gum disease, pain from sinuses or from ears.

Symptoms and signs: In tooth decay there is initially a sharp but short-lived pain. Later, severe and longer lasting pain occurs. Toothache pain is worst on eating or drinking. The person may also suffer from jaw ache, swollen face, loss of appetite, distress, emotional or behavioural changes, for example hand-flapping, shouting, head banging and biting, especially if they are unable to communicate their distress in any other way. Putting a hand to the face or a finger in the mouth is a common indication. The site of the toothache will be tender.

Investigations: These include dental assessment and x-ray of teeth.

Complications: Usually there are none, but the serious condition of bacterial endocarditis (Chapter 6) must be prevented.

Treatment: Painkillers (paracetamol), heat to the side of the face and use of gel may give temporary relief. The underlying cause must be treated.

Prevention of tooth disease

Good dental care involves a number of issues: understanding the need for good dental hygiene, daily brushing of teeth and gums, regular check-ups, early treatment for problems and a good diet to reduce sugar. The use of floss and fluoride therapy is essential to prevent decay. The person should be encouraged to eat fruit and vegetables rather than sweets and soft drinks, and to use mouthwashes and mouth rinses. People need regular support from a dental hygienist to remove scales and plaque. Disclosing tablets (food dye) may be used to disclose the plaque on teeth and as an aid to thorough cleaning.

The presence of heart disease or other health problems needs to be mentioned to the dentist. Antibiotics will need to be given prior to dental treatment if a heart lesion is present. Many people with Down syndrome are well supported by a mainstream dentist, however some people may need specialist support from a dentist experienced with working with people with a learning disability. Regular check-ups are important. Use of an electric toothbrush is recommended.

Tooth decay (Caries)

Tooth decay occurs mainly in young adults. Decay of the tooth root (exposed by shrinking of the gums) can be a problem in older people.

Causes: Plaques form due to bacterial action on saliva and food particles. Sugar in food is fermented and acid is formed which destroys enamel and over time leads to tooth decay. Sources of sugar include sweets, honey, fizzy drinks, fruit juices, fruit cordials, biscuits, cakes, frosted cereals, canned fruit, baked beans and salad cream.

Symptoms and signs/Investigations/Complications: (See toothache above). In the early stages there may be no pain.

Treatment and prevention: It is best to avoid sugary foods, especially as snacks between meals and just before going to bed. Brushing teeth with fluoride toothpaste makes the outer covering of teeth (enamel) more resistant to bacterial action. Early stages of tooth decay may be helped by the application of a fluoride varnish. In severe cases the decayed area will need to be removed and replaced with a filling and/or root canal treatment, or the person may need the tooth extracted.

Improper fitting together of upper and lower teeth (Malocclusions)

Causes: Missing teeth, small teeth, peg-shaped teeth are common for some people this can be made worse with tongue protrusion.

Symptoms and signs: These include poorly spaced teeth, the lower jaw too far back or too far forward, leading to over-biting.

Investigations: Investigation involves dental assessment with x-rays of teeth and the taking of tooth moulds.

Complications: Chewing food becomes difficult. There is an increased risk of tooth decay and gum disease.

Treatment: If the problem is severe orthodontic care is required. This can include the use of braces, retainers to help alignment and/or extraction of teeth.

Inflammation of the gums (Gingivitis)

This is common, often affecting the lower jaw front teeth and upper jaw back teeth.

Causes: It is often due to poor dental hygiene. Toxins produced by bacteria in dental plaque can irritate the gums and they become inflamed. It can also occur as the result of an impaired immune system.

Symptoms and signs: (See toothache above). These include tender and swollen gums, gums that bleed easily and bad breath. The person may avoid brushing their teeth.

Investigations: Dental assessment will be required.

Complications: Loss of teeth, formation of cysts (collections of fluids) or abscesses (collections of pus) can result. The serious condition of bacterial endocarditis (Chapter 6) is a possible complication.

Treatment: (See toothache above). If bleeding is noted during brushing, spend a little more time on the affected area. With careful and thorough removal of dental plaque the condition should resolve in about two weeks. If bleeding persists see the dentist. Use of a gel containing chlorhexidine (Corsodyl) may help.

Inflammation of gums around teeth (Periodontitis)

Causes: Toxins produced by plaque can damage the periodontal area and cause bone around the tooth to be lost. Periodontitis generally follows on as a natural progression from untreated gingivitis (above).

Symptoms and signs: In the early stages this condition is superficially indistinguishable from gingivitis (above). Over a period of time the tooth appears to become longer as the gums recede and as the root of the tooth is exposed, pain may be experienced when it is stimulated mechanically (tooth brushing), chemically (sugary foods) or thermally (hot or cold food). Halitosis (bad breath) is a common feature of periodontal disease. As bone is progressively destroyed the tooth becomes noticeably loose within the socket. Eventually so much of the support tissues are lost that chewing on the affected tooth/teeth becomes painful. At this stage hard food will be avoided in preference for soft. However, the affected tooth will often appear to be quite sound and undecayed. It is not unusual to find that the roots of the teeth in people with Down syndrome are shorter than usual. This can result in teeth becoming loose sooner than might otherwise be expected.

Complications: Periodontal abscesses (collections of pus) may develop. These bear a superficial resemblance to abscesses produced by tooth decay, being extremely painful and producing similar swellings. A serious condition of bacterial endocarditis (Chapter 6).

Investigations: Dental assessment is required.

Treatment: (See gingivitis above).

Grinding of teeth (Bruxism)

Causes: Often no specific cause is found. Known causes include anxiety, mood changes, dental malocclusions (above), and reduced facial muscle tone.

Symptoms and signs: Rhythmic grinding or clenching usually during sleep, but this can occur during the day.

Complications: These commonly include wearing down of the teeth, loosening of teeth, and stiffness of the jaw.

Treatment: Regular monitoring is required to check for complications. A biteplate/mouth guard may give some relief.

Chapter 13

Skin conditions

Skin, nail and hair problems may appear to be relatively minor in nature, but such problems can cause considerable unrecognised distress to individuals and to their family members and support workers. Skin problems are extremely common in adults with Down syndrome due to increased dry skin, impaired body immunity and reduced hygiene.

Spots (Acne)

Acne is very common. Spots often occur in areas of the face, back and chest, usually begin in puberty and are thought to be affected by the levels of sex hormones.

Causes: Blockage of hair/sweat ducts leads to build up of secretions. This condition can run in families, be caused by hormonal changes, the side-effect of medication (eg anti-convulsants, steroids), or the result of cosmetic creams. Associations with chocolate and salt are not supported by the evidence.

Symptoms and signs: Acne includes blackheads, whiteheads, cysts, boils and pimples. Spots can heal whilst others appear.

Investigations: If the acne is severe investigation needs to exclude an imbalance of sex hormones.

Complications: Picking or squeezing of spots can lead to scarring. Acne can cause social embarrassment and loss of self-esteem.

Treatment and prevention: Several treatments may be proposed but all have limited benefit. These include a change in diet, frequent washing and sunshine/ultraviolet light. Initially treatment is in the form of face washes; however if these do not help then oral tablets can be tried. Particular drugs for acne include benzoyl peroxide, antibiotics, retinoids, antiseborrheic medications, anti-androgen medications, hormonal treatments, salicylic acid, alpha hydroxyl acid, azelaic acid, nicotinamide, and keratolytic soaps. The oral contraceptive pill may be prescribed. Laser surgery has been used to reduce the scars left behind by acne. Usually acne settles over time.

Boils

An inflamed pus-filled area of skin, usually on the person's back, armpits, neck or groin. Boils can appear one at a time or several at a time.

Causes: Bacterial infection of the hair follicle which leads to a build up of pus under the skin.

Symptoms and signs: There is a painful, red, tender swelling with pus, which eventually heals to leave a scar.

Investigations: Diabetes should be excluded. If recurrent boils occur it may be necessary to swab the nose and armpits to detect a possible site harbouring bacteria.

Complications: Usually there are none.

Treatment and prevention: Simple measures such as gentle washing daily with antibacterial soap, drying area thoroughly and improving the immune system with vitamin C and zinc can be beneficial. When a lesion develops medical help will be needed to swab the area with antiseptic and possibly break the skin with a sterile needle to release the pus. A warm compress can help to remove pus. Antibiotics may be necessary to kill the bacteria together with skin anaesthetics ointments to reduce discomfort. Recurrent boils will require more intensive therapy. Infections from the boil can spread to other parts of the body or to others, so infected areas should not be touched.

Eczema (Atopic dermatitis)

This is a particular type of inflammation of the skin, more common in children. By teenage years the majority of people will be clear of the disease. Adult eczema usually involves the back of neck, elbows, wrists, ankles and knees.

Causes: Often there is no known cause, but it can be due to allergies, eg to a particular food. The person may also have asthma or hay fever. Eczema often runs in families.

Symptoms and signs: Commonly the person will have very dry skin which may be red, scaly, itchy, weepy and oozing. There is likely to be discomfort and excoriations (irritations, such as that caused by scratching, lesions). It can be exacerbated with heat, humidity, drying of skin and contact with clothes. Emotional and behavioural difficulties can occur.

Investigations: Usually none are required.

Complications: Secondary infections and thickening of skin can occur.

Treatment and prevention: Emollients (agents which soften skin, eg E45 and unguentum merck cream) can be applied to damp skin after bathing. The person needs to have warm, not hot, baths and to avoid use of perfumed soaps and wool clothing. The skin should be patted dry, not rubbed. Sunlight/ultraviolet light can help. Mild skin steroid creams (used sparingly and with caution), coal tar ointment, antibiotics, anti-histamine drugs (for itching) can be given. Specialist care from a dermatologist may be required.

Psoriasis
A chronic skin disease with thickened patches of inflamed red skin with a fluctuating course.

Causes: Often there is no known cause but it can be associated with a throat infection and made worse with emotional upset and trauma.

Symptoms and signs: There is reddened silvery scaled plaques, usually over the elbows, knees, and scalp. Finger-nails can become thickened and pitted. Itching is less than with eczema. Often there are symmetrical lesions over the body.

Investigations: Usually none are required.

Complications: Joint, scalp or nail involvement can occur.

Treatment and prevention: Emollient (substance to soften skin) cream, Dithranol, retinoids and steroid cream for the skin are the main forms of treatment. Ultraviolet light, sunbathing (with care) has been shown to be beneficial.

Seborrhoeic dermatitis
An inflammation of skin where there is a high area of sebaceous glands (glands of the body which produce oils), usually on the face, scalp, chest and back.

Causes: Unknown, but made worse by stress.

Symptoms and signs: These include flaking, redness, and pustules, scaly, itchy skin with a rash.

Investigations: Usually none are required.

Complications: Can spread to areas of face, eyebrows, nasal folds, ears.

Treatment and prevention: Avoid scratching and irritating substances. Shampoos with fungi static action can be of initial help. Use 3-7 times per week. Antibiotic or steroid creams can also be beneficial.

Xerosis

Dry, pale skin with poor elasticity.

Causes: Often the cause is unknown, but the condition is more common with increasing age.

Symptoms and signs: Skin is dry and cracked and can be itchy and scaly.

Investigations/Complications: Usually there are none.

Treatment and prevention: The person should avoid soaps which dry the skin and oils after bathing. Lubricating creams and creams to soften the skin may help. Showers should be warm, not hot. Cold dry weather should be avoided. Humidified air within the home can be beneficial.

Hair loss (Alopecia)

Causes: Often no cause is found, but alopecia might possibly be due to an autoimmune association (when the body's defences inappropriately respond against particular tissues or substance), or premature ageing. Severe stress, hormonal imbalance, drugs and iron deficiency can be known causes. Compulsive pulling of hair (trichotillomania) can be a cause.

Symptoms and signs: There can be patches of hair loss over any part of the body, but normally on the scalp, though it can include the beard, eyelashes and eyebrows. Hair may regrow or it may develop into total hair loss (Alopecia totalis).

Investigations: Underlying causes such as thyroid disease should be ruled out.

Complications: The condition can cause emotional and social difficulties.

Treatment: Active treatment is possible, but this will depend on the degree of concern caused to the person with Down syndrome and their family members by the hair loss. Small areas of hair loss can regrow without active treatment. Severe hair loss can be treated with medication under medical supervision. Large doses of steroids can improve regrowth, but a relapse is likely after the treatment is stopped. Side-effects from the medication are an important concern, eg weight gain, puffiness, and reduced appetite. Other drugs, such as minoxidil (Rogaine) have also been shown to be beneficial. Conservative management, eg wearing of a wig, may be appropriate and safer than active treatment.

Vitiligo
Areas of loss of pigmentation on the skin.

Causes: Often there is no obvious cause. Vitiligo occurs when melanocytes, the cells responsible for skin pigmentation, die or are unable to function. Occasionally it is due to thyroid disease, autoimmunity (body defences attack itself), old injuries or viral infections.

Symptoms and signs: Patches of well-defined areas of white skin can appear anywhere on body, more commonly on the hands, elbows, feet and face.

Investigations: An underlying condition should be excluded.

Complications: Affected areas are susceptible to sunburn and therefore must be covered or sun creams used. The condition can affect the person's confidence and self-esteem.

Treatment and prevention: Spontaneous improvement may occur. In mild cases, vitiligo can be masked with makeup or other cosmetic camouflage solutions. Steroid cream can be used with medical advice and caution. Particular forms of medication along with ultraviolet light may be considered (psoralen and ultraviolet A light (PUVA) treatment).

Cheilitis
Fissuring and crusting of lips with inflammation at corner of mouth.

Causes: Often no cause is found. Occasionally the condition is due to eczema, infections secondary to saliva collecting in corners of mouth or nutritional deficiencies.

Symptoms and signs: There is redness, scaling and itchiness around lips.

Investigations/Complications: Usually none are required.

Treatment: This includes moisturisation of lips, eg white petroleum, keep hydrated, using a humidifier and anti-fungal cream (Lotrimin) for infections. Any underlying cause should be treated.

Cutis marmorata and acrocyanosis
Discolouration of the skin. Commonly found in adults with Down syndrome.

Causes: Nerves and smaller blood vessels become sensitive to cold temperature.

Symptoms and signs: Cutis marmorata is a bluish mottling of the skin. Acrocyanosis is a cold-red decolourisation of the hands and feet.

Investigations: A medical assessment is required to exclude a serious blood circulation problem.

Treatment and prevention: Extremities of the body should be kept warm with increased clothing and heating.

Tinea pedis (athlete's foot)
Infection of the feet/toes.

Causes: Caused by a fungal infection, often due to poor drying between toes.

Symptoms and signs: There is scaling, cracking, itching and redness of toes. Blistering of the feet can occur.

Investigations: Usually none are required, but scrapings from feet can be examined for fungi.

Treatment: Feet should be kept dry. Foot powders with antifungal agent can be prescribed or potassium permanganate foot soaks, Miconazole powder or oral griseofulvin to treat fungus.

Onychomycosis
Infection of finger- and toe-nails.

Causes: Fungal infection

Symptoms and signs: Nails become opaque, white, thickened, friable or brittle.

Investigations: If the infection is severe clippings can be taken for analysis of the fungus.

Treatment and prevention: Antifungal medication is usually prescribed, eg griseofulvin. Therapy for several years may be required. Good nail care should be maintained, with frequent cutting of the toe-nails.

Chapter 14

Hormonal and blood-related issues

Hormones are chemicals produced by particular glands in the body specifically to have an effect on the function of one or more organs some distance away. The most important glands include the pituitary gland, the thyroid gland, adrenal glands, pancreas, ovaries (females) and testes (males) (Figure 11). Their action may be time-specific, eg on sexual maturation and on growth, or may occur throughout life, eg blood sugar control by insulin. The level of a hormone in the blood needs to be within certain limits, too much or too little can cause serious ill-health.

Blood contains a vast number of substances which play an important part in healthy bodily function. Such substances may be increased or decreased in quantity or be abnormal in shape or size. Regular screening of the levels of the blood substances is recommended for all persons with Down syndrome. A medical opinion should be sought if the person, the family or other carers have any concerns.

Hormones

Thyroid disorders

The thyroid gland is found in the front part of the neck (Figure 11). It produces a number of hormones, in particular two called thyroxine (T4) and tri-iodothyronine (T3), which help to maintain the body's metabolic rate and the function of proteins and nerve cells. The gland is principally under the control of another hormone 'thyroid stimulating hormone' (TSH) produced by the pituitary gland, a gland which serves to control and regulate many hormone producing glands. The thyroid gland can become overactive (hyperthyroidism) and speed up the body's metabolism or become underactive (hypothyroidism) and slow down the body's metabolism. Several combinations of high or low T4 and/or high or low T3 are possible. One-third of adults with Down syndrome have some evidence of a thyroid disorder.

Figure 11: **Glands of the human body**

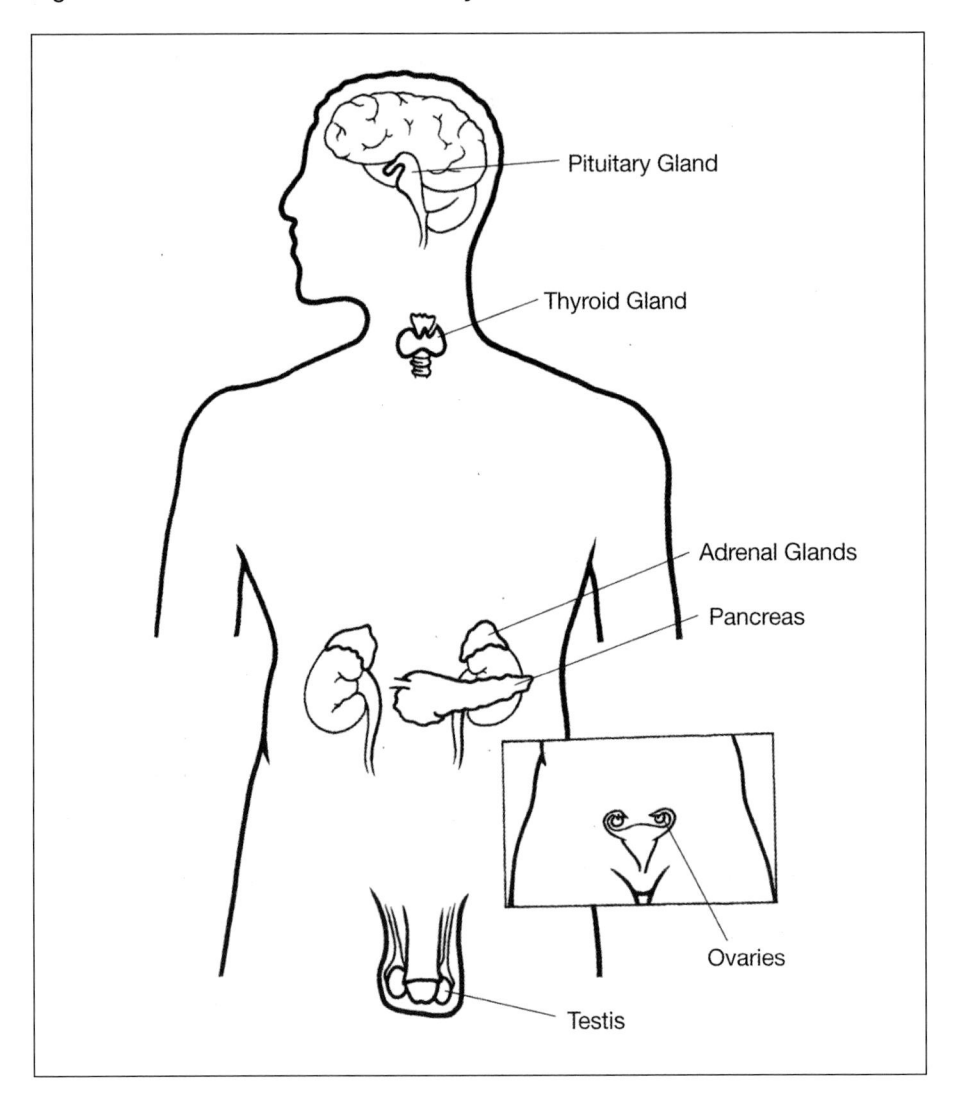

- Pituitary Gland
- Thyroid Gland
- Adrenal Glands
- Pancreas
- Ovaries
- Testis

Hypothyroidism

A condition where there is reduced activity of the thyroid gland. Associated low levels of the hormone thyroxine are found in the blood. This is the commonest thyroid disorder in adults with Down syndrome.

Causes: The condition can be present at birth. Birth hypothyroidism is uncommon and nowadays is detected by routine neonatal screening.

Acquired hypothyroidism is the development of an under activity of the thyroid gland during one's lifetime and is usually due to autoimmunity (the body's defence system attacks itself; this is also known as Hashimoto's Thyroiditis) or due to inflammation of the thyroid gland. The risk of developing hypothyroidism increases with age. Women are at a greater risk than men. Hypothyroidism can occasionally be due to medication (eg lithium), in areas with iodine deficiency in the diet or following surgery on the thyroid gland.

Symptoms and signs: Many symptoms can occur: slowing down, dry hair, weight gain, slow pulse, constipation, abnormal periods, mental deterioration, tiredness, heart failure, rough skin, loss of hair, deafness, anaemia, or early puberty.

Investigations: A diagnosis on appearance only can be difficult and blood tests are necessary. For hypothyroidism the blood level of the thyroid stimulating hormone is raised and the blood level of thyroxine is low. Antibodies (proteins produced by the body's immune system against the thyroid gland) may be present. If the thyroid gland is underactive due to lack of pituitary function, the TSH and thyroxine levels will be low.

Complications: Hypothyroidism can cause premature puberty, heart disease (Chapter 6) or present as a dementia related illness (Chapter 15).

Treatment and prevention: Thyroxine replacement therapy (a tablet or tablets taken every day) is necessary. The dose is increased depending on response and blood levels. Life-long therapy is often required. For borderline hypothyroidism (normal blood level of thyroxine, but raised level of thyroid stimulating hormone) monitoring is required if the person is asymptomatic. If symptomatic or thyroid antibodies are present, then the doctor will treat positively with thyroxine replacement. Routine screening is recommended – the minimum requirement is every two years. Other medications can affect thyroxine blood levels, eg lithium and iron tablets reduce blood thyroxine, whereas aspirin can increase thyroxine blood levels.

Hyperthyroidism
An overactive thyroid gland that leads to increased blood levels of thyroxine. It is less common than hypothyroidism.

Causes: This can include: autoimmunity 'Graves Disease' (the body's defence system attacks itself), an enlargement of the thyroid (a goitre or adeoma producing excess thyroxine), inflammation of thyroid gland or certain drugs. Sometimes no cause is found.

Symptoms and signs: Weight loss, increased appetite, behavioural change, tremor, diarrhoea, irritability, swelling of the thyroid gland, breathlessness, thinning hair, heat intolerance, bulging eyes and palpitations are all symptoms of hyperthyroidism.

Investigations: Blood tests are undertaken for thyroid hormone levels; low level of thyroid stimulating hormone, but high blood level of thyroxine. High blood levels of thyroid stimulating hormone and thyroxine imply a problem with the pituitary gland. Thyroid antibodies may be present.

Complications: Heart failure, behavioural or emotional changes are possible complications.

Treatment: Anti thyroid drugs (carbimazole) can be given to reduce the thyroid gland activity, surgery might be undertaken (thyroidectomy) or radioactive iodine given to reduce the function of the thyroid gland. The opinion of an endocrinologist (a specialist doctor in the management of hormonal disorders) is required. Hypothyroidism can develop after treatment.

Diabetes mellitus

A condition where there is a chronic high glucose level in the blood due to insulin deficiency or resistance to the action of insulin. Insulin is produced by the pancreas and is necessary for glucose to enter into cells; otherwise the glucose builds up in the blood.

Type I diabetes is an autoimmune condition where there is complete failure of the pancreas to produce any insulin.

Type 2 diabetes is when there is poor insulin production and increased resistance to insulin by the body's cells, it is related to obesity. It can be controlled by strict diet and oral drugs, but some people need insulin replacement treatment.

Causes: Type 1 diabetes is an autoimmune condition (the body's defence system attacks itself). In Type 2 diabetes there is a relationship to obesity and also some genetic predisposition.

Symptoms and signs: Commonly in Type 1 diabetes there is excessive urine output, thirst, weight change, skin infections, visual loss and behavioural changes. If diabetes is left untreated the person can develop 'diabetic ketoacidosis' with confusion and loss of consciousness, which can be life threatening.

Type 2 diabetes can be asymptomatic, but diabetes is often picked up at routine screening.

Investigations: Testing is undertaken for a high blood glucose level (even after fasting), glucose and proteins in urine. If borderline, a further 'glucose tolerance test' can be done to see how the body responds to a high level of sugar.

Complications: These can include 'hypoglycaemic attacks' commonly after too much insulin, sickness or alcohol and there is too little glucose in blood. This presents with weakness, confusion, sweating, pallor and dizziness. Treatment is to quickly increase the sugar in the blood, eg by sugary drinks, sweets, glucose tablets. If the person is unable to swallow then medical attention should be obtained for glucose to be given intravenously.

High levels of glucose in the blood (usually due to poor compliance with insulin) can lead to 'diabetic ketoacidosis', a serious medical condition which presents with a 'fruity-smelling breath', loss of appetite, nausea, vomiting, stomach pains, coma. Long-term problems associated with diabetes include hypertension, poor circulation, heart disease, eye disease including cataracts, kidney and nerve damage and recurrent infections.

Treatment: In Type 1 diabetes insulin injections and strict monitoring of carbohydrate intake is always required as the body has no way of producing insulin. Weight and diet monitoring can control type 2 diabetes initially. However often this is insufficient and therefore diabetic drugs which try to stimulate further insulin or reduce insulin resistance are needed. If this is unsuccessful insulin injections are required. Advice from a dietician and a specialist doctor in the treatment of diabetes is necessary for people whose condition is complex. Careful measuring of diabetic control is required including urine tests for glucose and proteins, blood tests for glucose level and the substance called 'glycosylated haemoglobin (Hgb AIC)' which gives a measure of the average level of blood glucose over the last 8-10 weeks. Careful monitoring and support is needed to prevent serious complications, particularly diabetic retinopathy and foot ulcers. Most people with diabetes should undertake regular screening for these conditions. Advice and support to the person concerned and anyone supporting them, is important. Immediate medical help must always be sought if severe complications occur.

Gout
A metabolic disorder affecting the joints.

Causes: There are increased blood levels of uric acid which lead to arthritis (usually in one joint). The big toe is the most common joint affected, but it can also affect the knee, ankle, wrist, and hands.

Symptoms and signs: Commonly the joint is red, swollen, tender and very painful. Joint pain usually begins during the night. The person may have several attacks.

Investigations: A blood test is undertaken to find out if there is a high blood uric acid, x-ray of the joint to show any inflammation and removal of fluid from the joint to test for uric acid crystals.

Complications: There can be arthritis in the joint. Recurrent attacks are not uncommon.

Treatment and prevention: The person should drink plenty of fluids. Non-steroidal anti-inflammatory drugs (aspirin, naproxen), or colchicines may be prescribed to reduce pain. Blood levels of uric acid can be lowered with other drugs (allopurinol or probenecid) which are given after the acute attack has settled and are useful for preventing further episodes of gout. Drinks with high uric acid levels should be avoided.

Growth hormone
This is a hormone which is produced by the pituitary gland that stimulates normal body growth. To assess growth correctly charts designed specifically for children and young people with Down syndrome should be used because they may have an altered growth hormone metabolism. There is controversy in relation to whether children with Down syndrome may benefit from growth hormone replacement therapy. Adults are unlikely to benefit from growth hormone replacement (Chapter 2).

Sex hormones
Sex hormone tests measure levels of the sex hormones, including oestrogen, progesterone and testosterone. Tests are helpful to determine if secretion of these sex hormones is within normal levels. Several different types of tests are used to help diagnose numerous disorders and to monitor pregnancy. Few detailed studies have been reported for adults with Down syndrome. Generally for men the sex hormone testosterone is at a normal level. For women sex hormones may be at a normal or increased level.

Blood diseases

A number of blood disorders are associated with Down syndrome although the underlying mechanisms for such findings remain unresolved. **Serious medical complications can result if not treated. A medical opinion should always be sought if there is any concern.**

Anaemia

A decrease in the level of haemoglobin in the blood or decrease in number of red blood cells (RBCs).

Causes: Several causes are possible. The three main classes include excessive blood loss (acutely such as a haemorrhage or chronically through low-volume loss, eg heavy periods), excessive blood cell destruction (hemolysis) or deficient red blood cell production (bone marrow disease). Specific causes include reduced intake of vitamins required to make blood cells, which leads to iron deficiency (due to blood loss or insufficient intake of iron), vitamin B7 deficiency (if due to poor absorption in stomach called 'pernicious anaemia'), folic acid deficiency, or bone marrow disease (see aplastic anaemia below).

Symptoms and signs: These can often be absent or missed. Usually include fatigue, headaches, dizziness, fainting, breathlessness, pallor and a fast heart rate. Heart failure, behavioural and emotional changes can occur.

Investigations: The level of haemoglobin and number and size of RBCs in the blood should be measured. If these are low, tests are needed to determine the type of anaemia and underlying cause. Blood tests can be undertaken to measure the level of important vitamins and minerals in the blood (iron, B12, folic acid). If necessary, tests may be needed to determine level of other blood cells, eg white cell count, platelets. If these are also abnormal, investigations will be needed to examine the production of these by the bone marrow (bone marrow aspiration where a needle is inserted into the bone and a small amount of tissue is removed). Examination of a stained blood smear using a microscope can also be helpful to show the shape and size of the RBCs.

Complications: Heart failure is a possible complication (Chapter 6) and this can present as dementia (Chapter 15).

Treatment and prevention: These depend on the underlying cause. Generally an increase in the dietary intake of iron (eg red meat) and vitamins will treat the anaemia. Iron tablets (ferrous sulphate) and vitamin B12 injections can be prescribed if a change in the diet is not adequate. A blood transfusion is required only rarely. If either haemolysis or bone marrow disease is found, specialist input will be required.

Aplastic anaemia
Reduced number of red cells, white cells and platelets in the blood.

Causes: Abnormality in the normal function of the bone marrow exists due to autoimmunity (a condition where the body's own defence system attacks itself).

Symptoms and signs: (see anaemia above) There is increased risk of infections, bruising and bleeding.

Investigations: The level of the different cells in the blood should be measured. A bone marrow biopsy or a bone marrow aspiration (needle inserted into the bone and small amount of tissue removed) may be necessary.

Complications: Leukaemia (below) may result, but only rarely. If untreated, the condition is life threatening.

Treatment: The person will require blood transfusions, immuno-suppression drugs (strong drugs which can reduce the body's immune function) and a bone marrow transplant may be necessary. Day-to-day care is required to treat any bleeding and infections which may occur.

Polycythemia
An increase in the blood concentration of haemoglobin, volume or number of red blood cells.

Causes: Often the cause is unknown. The condition can be present at birth, or be secondary to heart disease (Chapter 6), bone marrow disorder, infection, trauma, bleeding or generally low oxygen in blood.

Symptoms and signs: These include headaches, reddened (plethoric) skin, blurred vision, hypertension, tiredness, circulatory problems and gout.

Investigations: Blood tests are necessary to find out the haemoglobin level and the number of red blood cells in the blood. The size of the red blood cells and the thickness of the blood must also be measured, as must other blood products such as white cells and platelets, which can also be raised. A bone marrow aspiration (removal of a sample of the inner part of some bone marrow) is sometimes undertaken.

Complications: The development of a blood clot, a stroke or heart disease can occur.

Treatment: Cells from the blood must be removed by venesection (procedure where blood is taken from a vein – similar to a blood donation) to 'thin' the blood. Medication can be used to stop the body producing red cells. Aspirin or anti-coagulation can be given to reduce the risk of developing a blood clot.

Neutropenia

Condition where there is a low blood count of some white cells called 'neutrophils'. Common finding in adults with Down syndrome and usually indicates no serious underlying problem.

Causes: The cause can be unknown, but may include a viral infection, rheumatoid arthritis or bone marrow disease. It can also be caused by drugs (eg chlorpromazine, immuno-suppressants, chemotherapy or radiotherapy).

Symptoms and signs: There is increased risk of infections.

Investigations: Usually none is required. If the condition is severe then the number of white blood cells in the blood can be measured and a bone marrow aspiration undertaken (removal of a sample of the inner part of the bone with a needle) to detect the presence of any underlying disease.

Complications: These will be secondary to any infection.

Treatment: Antibiotics can be prescribed if the person is unwell. General good hygiene is important – antiseptic mouthwashes for example. If medication is the cause it should be changed. If a fever develops, this can be a medical emergency and advice should be sought early.

Leukaemia

Cancer of the white blood cells. There are different types of leukaemia. Some can be for a short period and often more aggressive (acute); others progress slowly and there is deterioration over several years (chronic). Common types include acute lymphoblastic leukaemia (ALL) and acute myeloid leukaemia (AML).

Causes: These are unknown although some predisposing genes have been found. The condition is seen more often in children than in adults with Down syndrome.

Symptoms and signs: These include tiredness, fever, infections, pain in joints, bleeding, stomach pains, swollen abdomen, pallor, bruising, enlarged liver or spleen and swollen glands.

Investigations: Diagnosis is confirmed by measuring the number of white blood cells in the blood and in the bone marrow by a bone marrow aspiration (needle inserted into the bone to obtain a piece of bone marrow). Often these cells are very immature and do not function well. A lumbar puncture (procedure where fluid is removed from the spine), CT/MRI scan may be undertaken to determine the spread of the disease.

Complications: Leukaemia can lead to serious ill-health and in severe cases is life threatening.

Treatment: Treatment from a specialist oncology (cancer) service is important. Initially blood transfusions are used to improve symptoms (of red blood cells and platelets necessary to maintain a high level of normal cells in blood). To try and cure the disease chemotherapy involving drugs and radiotherapy to kill cancer cells is usually necessary. There are a number of complications associated with these forms of therapy, including a proneness to infections, a resultant high blood sugar level and ulcers in the mouth or in the bowel. There is a good outlook for ALL, but less good for AML. Family support is important. Bone marrow transplantation can be considered.

Myelofibrosis

An increased fibrosity of the bone marrow. Inability of the bone marrow to produce normal blood cells.

Causes: The cause is unknown, but myelofibrosis can be part of leukaemia.

Symptoms and signs/Investigations: (See anaemia above).

Complications: There can be recurrent infections, hypertension, blood clots, leukaemia. The condition can be life threatening.

Treatment: Blood transfusions are often required. Treatment should be given for any underlying cause and infections.

Macrocytosis
An increase in the size of the red blood cells, a common abnormality in people with Down syndrome.

Causes: Usually there is no serious underlying cause and the condition reflects the early release of red blood cells from the bone marrow. Known causes include vitamin B12 (folate) or thyroid deficiency. There is a possible association with premature ageing and Alzheimer's disease (Chapter 15).

Symptoms and signs: These are secondary to the cause.

Investigations: These include assessing blood cell count and size of red blood cells MCV (mean corpuscular volume), and measuring vitamin B12, folic acid and thyroid hormone levels.

Complications: These are secondary to the cause.

Treatment: If there is no underlying cause which requires treatment then the condition just needs to be monitored on a regular basis.

Transient myeloproliferative disorder
A condition similar to leukaemia, but present for a brief time and not requiring treatment. However a proportion of those affected can develop leukaemia later on.

Immune system and immunisations

The immune system protects the body from invading organisms such as bacteria and viruses. It does this by a number of means, but primarily by producing antibodies (proteins produced by the body's immune system which help to neutralise infecting agents such as bacteria or viruses), and by activating white blood cells. Invaders are first recognised, then killed. Most importantly the makeup of the invader is remembered so that a further infection is readily dealt with. Some people with Down syndrome have a problem with their immune system leading to frequent and recurrent infections, cancers and the condition in which parts of their own body are attacked as if they were invaders (autoimmunity). The most common problems are reduction in some white cells (neutropenia) and an increase in autoimmunity (especially thyroid autoimmunity). A high rate of Hepatitis B virus carriers has been reported (Chapter 8).

Generally, if an adult with Down syndrome is well, there is no reason why they cannot have the regular immunisations that are given to the general population. Tetanus-diphtheria, influenza, pneumonia, chickenpox, Hepatitis B should be considered and given by the person's GP.

Chapter 15

Psychological, emotional and mental health issues

Emotional and psychological wellbeing is important to everyone. For adults with Down syndrome, as for others, there is undoubtedly a complex interaction between genetic, physical, psychological, social and environmental factors which affect mental and physical health and wellbeing. An emotional difficulty often has an impact on other areas of the person's life.

Like other people, adults with Down syndrome may experience psychological and emotional difficulties and mental health issues. Some of these may relate to other people's perceptions of them and behaviour towards them, treating them like children rather than adults with the same rights and needs as everyone else. This may mean they are denied the opportunities to grow and develop as adults with the right to make decisions about their own lives (with support if necessary) and the chance to take reasonable, assessed risks.

The accurate diagnosis and treatment of psychological and emotional problems is important for both physical and mental health. However, making the correct diagnosis may be difficult because of the person's underlying cognitive impairments (particularly of communication), compounding medical conditions (eg sensory loss), poor test compliance and a lack of knowledge by professionals regarding what is 'normal' and what is not for people with Down syndrome. In the same way as for physical conditions, any concerns regarding emotional difficulties and mental health should lead to an informed opinion from a professional with an understanding of the relevant area of health care for adults with Down syndrome.

Sleep disturbance

This is common and may involve a problem in falling asleep, waking during the night, waking early or sleeping at inappropriate times of the day.

Causes: There may be no apparent reason, but it can be part of depression, anxiety disorder, physical condition, dementia or be due to the side-effects of medication.

Symptoms and signs: There might be problems with settling, waking at night, restless sleep, rituals, refusing to go to bed or snoring loudly. Secondary problems include feeling tired, less happy, irritable, hyperactive, anxious, having poor concentration and memory and under-performing in day-to-day activities.

Investigations: Underlying physical or psychological causes such as depression, anxiety or sleep apnoea should be ruled out.

Complications: These might include daytime behavioural changes.

Treatment and prevention: Simple measures may help, such as a routine sleep programme, relaxation, reduced caffeine intake, exercise and a warm bath. A behavioural programme with minimal fuss and a set procedure at night with advice and support from a community nurse can be beneficial. Melatonin (naturally occurring brain hormone) can be prescribed. Hypnotic medication (eg zopiclone, lorazepam) can be given but is best avoided or used for a few days only. Low dose antidepressants (eg trazadone, amitriptyline) or antihistamines with sedation properties can benefit some individuals.

Bereavement
A physical and/or emotional response in the months following the death of someone close. Reactions vary from person to person and are dependent on whether the death was sudden or after long illness, the closeness of the relationship, whether the person was told about the death in a way that they could understand and the subsequent support provided. All aspects of the person's wellbeing may be affected – emotional, physical, spiritual and social – but the overriding feeling is one of intense pain or grief in missing someone.

Causes: Loss of a close relationship.

Symptoms and signs: These can include: a sense of shock, numbness, grief, guilt, depression, behavioural changes, disturbed sleep, self-harm, hollowness in the stomach, over-sensitivity to noise, tightness in the chest or throat, lack of energy, fatigue and breathlessness, anxiety, loneliness, helplessness, hopelessness, shock, numbness and yearning for the dead person, appetite disturbances, absent-minded behaviour, social withdrawal, dreams of the deceased, avoiding reminders of the deceased, sighing, restless overactivity, crying, confusion, preoccupation with the deceased, a sense of presence of the deceased, auditory and visual hallucinations.

Complications: There may be prolonged bereavement reaction, depressive illness, and severe changes in behaviour.

Treatment: Support from others and counselling are the mainstay of appropriate management of the grief and loss which accompany bereavement. Such support allows the person, over time, to come to accept their loss and to manage their grief. Mild tranquillisers can help sleep and any disturbed behaviour. Anti-depressants can be prescribed if the bereavement process is thought to be not resolving or there is evidence of depression (see below). For more information on bereavement support see appendices D and E.

Delirium

This is a state of acute confusion that is more common in older adults with Down syndrome or those with physical ill-health.

Causes: Delirium can be caused by many disorders including a physical illness, infections, high fever, side-effects of drugs, drug toxicity, metabolic disturbances and epilepsy (Chapter 11).

Symptoms and signs: There may be confusion, clouding of awareness, anxiety, restlessness, mood swings, illusions (misinterpretation of real objects, eg sees spots on curtains as spiders), hallucinations (experience of something being present when not there in reality, eg a feeling of spiders crawling over body, but no spiders are present), bizarre ideas, violence and inattention, all of which can be worse at night.

Investigations: Investigations should be undertaken to find the underlying cause, including blood screen, evidence of urine infection, drug levels or more intensive tests (eg MRI/CT brain scan).

Complications: Injuries may result from delirium. Other complications are secondary to underlying cause. If not treated the condition may prove life threatening.

Treatment: The underlying cause should be treated and anxiety reduced. Clear lighting is important and fluid intake should be maintained. The person may require admission to hospital and tranquillising medication (eg chlorpromazine, haloperidol).

Depression
This is a psychological condition of persistently feeling sad with a loss of interest in day-to-day activities. Most people feel mildly depressed at certain times during their lives, often as a reaction to a situation, but this is usually short-lived.

Causes: Often there is no apparent reason, but it can commonly be a result of the loss of someone close, the presence of a physical illness, a major life change or the side-effects of medication.

Symptoms and signs: These include: a depressed mood, crying for no reason, loss of interest, reduced energy, tiredness, weight loss or gain, disturbed sleep pattern, reduced activity or agitation, negative thoughts, guilt, poor concentration, disturbed memory, diminished appetite, decline in social skills, occasionally thoughts of self-harm, loss of confidence, behavioural changes, delusions (irrational ideas, eg the postman trying to poison them) and hallucinations (experience of something being present when not there in reality, eg feeling of spiders crawling over body, but no spiders present). Episodes may recur or be associated with episodes of feeling 'high'. Physical complaints (eg abdominal pain, stopping of periods, headaches) can occur. There may be a decline in daily self-care skills and social skills.

Investigations: Depression should be differentiated from a physical problem, eg hypothyroidism or from some other psychological problem, eg bereavement, dementia (below).

Complications: These can include injury to others, self-harm, neglect and deterioration in physical health. There is an increased risk of further episodes and suicide (rare in adults with Down syndrome).

Treatment: Any underlying factors need to be managed. Depressive illness can be treated with behavioural therapy, counselling, and/or a course of antidepressants (group of drugs used to treat depression, eg amitriptyline, fluoxetine, lofepramine). Electroconvulsive therapy (ECT – form of treatment using seizures induced by electric shocks) can be used to treat people whose symptoms are severe. Individuals may not fully recover to their previous level of abilities. Antidepressant treatment may continue for many months to prevent future episodes of depression.

Dementia (Alzheimer's disease)
Dementia is a syndrome resulting from a disturbance of brain function, usually chronic and progressive, in which there is deterioration in memory, thinking, comprehension, language and learning. Other features include emotional change, deterioration in social behaviour and physical health. Alzheimer's disease and dementia are very common in older adults (50 years and over) with Down syndrome.

Causes: For older persons with Down syndrome, Alzheimer's disease is virtually always the cause of the dementia. Alzheimer's dementia is associated with large amounts of amyloid deposits (starch-like material) throughout the brain and neurofibrillary tangles (strands of protein) seen within the brain cells. The average age of onset of dementia in adults with Down syndrome is in the fifth decade, but it can begin as early as the third decade. Risk increases with age. Other causes of 'reversible' dementia-like symptoms include hypothyroidism (Chapter 14), depression (above), a physical illness, vitamin deficiency or the side-effects of medication. Recently incidences of Lewy-body dementia (dementia with features of Parkinson's disease with particular changes in the brain called 'Lewy bodies') and vascular dementia (dementia due to bleeding or blockage of brain blood vessels) have been reported in adults with Down syndrome.

Symptoms and signs: In the initial phase there may be memory impairment, disorientation in time, personality change, reduced speech output, apathy, behavioural changes, inattention and reduced social interactions. Later problems include loss of self-help skills such as dressing, toileting, feeding, walking often becomes slow and shuffling, hallucinations (experience of something being present when not there in reality) and delusions (irrational ideas) are possible. Late stage dementia is characterised by an inability to walk, choking episodes, being bed-ridden, incontinence, having a flexed posture, stiffness, jerking and seizures.

Investigations: It is important to assess for causes of decline other than dementia: for example is the decline part of the normal ageing process or is there a physical cause, eg hearing or vision impairment, delirium, the effects of medication, brain tumour, hypothyroidism or vitamin deficiency? A psychological cause also needs to be considered, eg depression, bereavement or a change in residence. Recent evidence would suggest that doctors can test for particular genes (apolipoprotein E genes) which influence the risk of a person developing Alzheimer's disease. Brain scans can show shrinkage of the brain.

Complications: These can include wandering, accidents, depression (above), and epilepsy (Chapter 11). Life-expectancy is significantly reduced. Dementia usually leads to death within 5-10 years after the onset of memory loss.

Treatment and prevention: Management by a specialist with knowledge of dementia in adults with learning disability is essential. Maintaining a familiar environment and a daily routine for as long as possible will help. Any underlying cause should be treated, eg hypothyroidism, depression. Particular problems, eg poor sleep, challenging behaviours can be treated with behavioural therapy preferably, though medication might be considered if strictly necessary. Support is essential to reduce stress. Social services, community learning disability nurses and carer organisations are important sources of help and support. The risk of accidents in the home should be assessed, eg dangers from fires, kitchen utensils etc. If transfer to a nursing or residential unit is necessary the situation needs to be handled with sensitivity and understanding. Recently donepezil (Aricept), rivastigamine (Exelon), galantamine (Reminyl) and memantine (Ebixa) are drugs which have been licensed to treat Alzheimer's disease in the general population. These drugs mainly enhance one of the chemicals (acetylcholine) in the brain. Benefit for people with Down syndrome who have dementia and who have been treated with these drugs has been reported.

No specific treatment is available to prevent dementia although numerous research studies have been undertaken. General good health may prevent the onset of dementia, eg keeping mentally active, doing exercise, having a good diet, no hypertension, diabetes or smoking. The role of anti-oxidants, eg vitamin E, non-steroidal anti-inflammatory drugs (aspirin), nutrients and the development of a vaccine remain controversial. Appendices D and E suggest sources of information and support.

Anxiety disorders

Can be a panic attack (periodic episodes of severe anxiety which is not restricted to a particular situation – sudden intense panic) or of a generalised anxiety type (persistent anxiety not restricted to any one situation).

Causes: No one particular factor accounts for anxiety attacks, but they can be due to a combination of genetic makeup, personality and the environment. Individuals with autism are more susceptible to anxiety attacks.

Symptoms and signs: These are numerous, including unpleasant feelings, fear of dying, feeling unreal, nervousness, dizziness, choking, sweating, trembling, palpitations, muscular tension, stomach discomfort, diarrhoea, behavioural changes, hyperactivity, irritability, aggression, looking strained and tense, over-breathing. Panic attacks can lead to social isolation and withdrawal.

Investigations: Screening for physical disorders should be undertaken, eg hyperthyroidism or hypoglycaemia (Chapter 14) and assessment for depression (above) and to ensure symptoms are not due to the side-effects of medication or as part of medication withdrawal. The type of anxiety disorder should be determined.

Complications: These can include depression, injuries (self or others), and behavioural changes and the condition can have a marked impact on the person's social relationships.

Treatment and prevention: Reassurance, counselling, relaxation and behavioural therapy can have a beneficial effect. Medication (mild tranquillisers, beta-blockers, antidepressants) can be prescribed but should be done under supervision and for a limited period only. Support and advice for carers is an important part of management.

Phobias

Condition where severe anxiety is provoked by a well-defined situation or object. Factors are often avoided or dreaded. Contemplation of factors can lead to anxiety. Specific phobias include heights, thunder and animals.

Causes/Symptoms and signs/Investigations/Complications/Treatment: (See anxiety disorders above).

Obsessive-compulsive disorder (OCD)

Recurrent persistent thoughts (obsessions) or repetitive rituals (compulsive acts). Thoughts may relate to ideas, images, impulses and actions. Behaviours are repeated again and again. The person is unable to resist and feels compelled to repeat the thoughts and/or actions causing distress. The condition is often chronic.

Causes: Often the cause is unknown but it can be associated with anxiety and depression.

Symptoms and signs: These commonly include repetitive thoughts, compulsive acts of washing, cleaning, checking, tidiness and excessive ordering. If the person tries to resist he/she becomes anxious. Serious disruption in day-to-day living occurs. The person can spend hours on the same compulsion.

Investigations: OCD needs to be differentiated from repetitive behaviours associated with the person's learning disability and an associated depressive illness or dementia (above) excluded.

Complications: OCD can lead to depression. Considerable stress can occur for the person, family members and support staff.

Treatment: Behavioural therapy, antidepressants (especially clomipramine, fluoxetine, paroxetine) can be of benefit, but the outcome is often poor. Support for the person concerned, family members and paid staff remains an important part of the management plan.

Mania/Hypomania
Psychological condition with disturbance of mood and associated overactivity, elation or irritability.

Causes: Often there is no obvious cause. It can be secondary to treatment with antidepressants or following environmental stress. A family history of the illness may be present.

Symptoms and signs: There are many features including elevated or irritable mood, increased energy and activity, sleep disturbance, excessive talking, overactivity, sexual indiscretions, distractibility, feelings of wellbeing and over familiarity. Disruption in daily living skills usually occurs. Hallucinations (experience of something being present when not) and delusions (irrational ideas) can occur. Aggression and behavioural changes are not uncommon.

Investigations: Screen for a medical condition should be undertaken, eg hyperthyroidism, delirium state. The condition should be differentiated from other mental health disorders, eg schizophrenia, dementia.

Complications: Physical injury or involvement in criminal behaviour can occur.

Treatment and prevention: Hospital care may be necessary. Tranquillising medication, eg risperidone, amisulpride, haloperidol may be required. The prevention of future relapse may be possible with long-term therapy with lithium, Depakote or carbamazepine medication.

Schizophrenia

A form of mental illness characterised by disturbance in thinking, emotion and behaviour. An uncommon condition which can be difficult to diagnose in people with a learning disability. The condition usually presents for longer than six months. Recurrent episodes can occur leading to chronic ill-health.

Causes: The cause is often unknown.

Symptoms and signs: These commonly include personality change, hallucinations (experience of something being present when not), delusions (irrational ideas), incoherent thought, disturbance of mood, abnormal behaviour, social isolation and the impairment of self-care skills. A feeling that others are sharing their thoughts, feelings or actions may be expressed by more able individuals. Onset can be slow and insidious. Recurrent episodes may lead to a 'negative state' of marked apathy, reduced speech, flat emotions and social withdrawal. Predominant symptoms may include marked paranoid ideas (abnormal ideas of persecution), aggression or changes in behaviour.

Investigations: Assessment should be undertaken for other causes of confusion, eg delirious state, epilepsy, depression, mania.

Complications: This can become a chronic condition. Recurrent relapses are common. Injury to self or to others may occur. It can occasionally lead to criminal offences, eg fire-setting, assaults on others.

Treatment: The person may require treatment in hospital. Antipsychotic medication (eg risperidone, amisulpride, and chlorpromazine) is often required. Support for the person concerned, family members and paid staff is important. Voluntary support groups are available. Compliance with medication is important to prevent a future relapse. Behavioural therapy can have a limited benefit. Ongoing community rehabilitation with the help of a community nurse and/or an occupational therapist is necessary for people whose condition is chronic.

Autistic spectrum conditions

In medical and psychological terms autism is classified as a developmental rather than a psychological condition. However it will be discussed here due to the psychological issues associated with the condition. People with autism will experience problems associated with their condition in relation to social interaction, communication, sensory issues and restricted repetitive behaviour.

The symptoms of autism are often manifest at an early age (usually before three years) although some people are not diagnosed until much later.

Causes: The cause, or causes, of autism are still not known although research is being undertaken to provide some indications. There is a growing body of evidence on the nature of the 'autistic' brain, the potential genetic predisposition to autism and certain genes that may increase susceptibility to autism. Reseach is complicated by the possibility that autism is not a single condition which emerges in a spectrum of forms, but rather a range of developmental conditions of the brain.

Investigations: Most people are diagnosed with an autistic spectrum condition in childhood by a specialist such as a child psychologist or paediatrician; they need to differentiate between behaviours associated with a learning disability, hearing or visual impairment, and from mental health difficulties such as depression or obsessive compulsive disorder (above).

Symptoms and signs: These can include in children: impaired social interaction (lack of response to others, impaired play activity, difficulties with make-believe), poor language expression and conversation, lack of gestures, restricted repertoire of activities and interests, repetitive behaviour, preference for a rigid routine, resistance to change and a preference for predictability. The person may be preoccupied with a special interest such as dates, routes, timetables, twiddling ribbons and strings etc. Other issues can include fears or phobias, sleep and eating problems, aggression and behaviour that is seen as challenging.

Complications: People with autism have an increased risk of other conditions. The National Autistic Society (see Appendix E for details) says that at least 70% of people with autism have an additional condition, eg epilepsy, bowel problems or mental health needs.

Treatment: Autism is a lifelong condition that affects each individual differently for their entire life. People need to be supported by others who understand their autism and treat them in a person centred way, recognising their unique personality, family and community situation. Positive behavioural support, advice for family members and paid staff and providing predictable support are recommended. With caution and close supervision, medication may be prescribed for some behaviours, eg risperidone for aggressive behaviour, Depakote for mood swings and propranolol for anxiety attacks.

Hyperkinetic Disorder (Attention Deficit Disorder or ADD)
Strictly speaking a hyperkinetic disorder is a disorder of development rather than of the mind. However there is a major emotional aspect to the condition as well as difficulties in behaviour. The disorder may be under-reported due to difficulty in distinguishing the disorder from the person's learning disability or from autism.

Causes: (See autistic spectrum conditions above).

Symptoms and signs: These can include: being overactive, fidgetiness, distractibility, impatience, inattentiveness, impulsivity, failure to complete activities, inability to follow instructions, poor listening. It can lead to difficulties with relationships and behaviour that is seen as challenging.

Investigations: It should be differentiated from other behavioural disorders; mood or anxiety problems and physical causes such as hyperthyroidism should be ruled out.

Complications: Behaviours seen as challenging can persist and there may be injuries to self or others.

Treatment: Treatment can include behavioural therapy, often with home and day care, and the avoidance of overstimulation. Psycho-stimulant drugs which stimulate the mind (eg Ritalin) can be used but only under close medical supervision.

Appendices and resources

Appendix A

Glossary of additional medical terms

Adenoids	The adenoids, also known as pharyngeal tonsils, are a mass of tissue which fights infections situated at the back of the nasal cavity where the nose blends into the throat.
Aortic coarctation	Is a condition found at birth where the aorta narrows near where it joined other heart vessels.
Atrial septal defect	Form of 'hole in the heart' heart defect at birth that enables blood flow between two compartments of the heart called the left and right atria.
Eustachian tube	Is a tube that links the top of the throat to the middle ear.
Grommets	Grommets are tiny plastic tubes that are inserted into the ear drum. They help equalise the pressure in the ear so the person can hear properly again.
Hysterectomy	Is the surgical removal of the uterus, usually performed by a gynaecologist.
Intelligence Quotient (IQ)	Is a score derived from one of several tests designed to assess intelligence. Average score is 100 and approximately 95% of the population score between 70 and 130.
Patent ductus arteriosus	Failure of the child's major blood vessel (called ductus arteriosus) to close normally after birth leading to mixing of blood near the heart. Can lead to heart failure.
Polycythemia	Is a disease state in which the proportion of blood volume that is occupied by red blood cells increases. It is often due to an increase in the number of red blood cells.
Thyroxine hormone	Produced by a gland in the neck the thyroid gland that is primarily responsible for regulation of body metabolism.
Thyroid stimulating hormone	Is a hormone that stimulates the thyroid gland to produce thyroxine. Released from the pituitary gland in the brain.
Ventricular septal defect	Is a defect ('hole in the heart') in the heart wall dividing the left and right ventricles of the heart.

Appendix B

Medical checklist

More so than for the general population it is important that individuals with Down syndrome receive the usual health care screening procedures and have regular health care check-ups to detect any possible illness. This applies to all adults with Down syndrome regardless of their age.

Below is a check list summarising the health issues, discussed in earlier chapters, which should be routinely assessed in adults with Down syndrome. A detailed medical history and a physical and psychological examination are the basis of a good health assessment. Particular attention should be given to some of the problems listed below. If health problems occur then a medical opinion should always be considered.

Particular problems for family members and support staff to watch out for:

- obesity
- decline in vision
- loss of hearing
- dental problems
- delayed sexual development
- problems with menstruation
- heart failure
- behavioural difficulties
- sleep apnoea
- depression
- dementia
- seizures

Particular health areas for professionals to observe:

- weight
- eyes (visual acuity, cataracts, keratoconus)
- ears (hearing loss)
- heart murmur
- sexual awareness development
- menstrual cycle
- epilepsy
- dental hygiene
- thyroid disease
- depression
- dementia
- behavioural difficulties
- medication

Routine checks family members, support staff and professionals should be aware of:

- measure weight at least once a year
- vision every 1-2 years
- hearing every 1-2 years
- teeth every 1-2 years
- thyroid function tests every 2-3 years
- blood sugar and cholesterol
- blood screen every 2-3 years
- breast and testicular examination monthly
- echocardiogram if heart murmur develops (exclude mitral valve prolapse)
- psychological status every 1-2 years
- review of medication every year
- urinalysis
- immunisations

Areas of further intervention by family members, support workers and professionals:

- education regarding health issues
- advice regarding particular health issues, eg dental care, obesity, hypothyroidism, epilepsy parent/carer support groups
- recreational/vocational programmes
- self-advocacy
- sex education
- consent issues
- how to access health and social services
- available residential facilities
- bereavement counselling for those who experience loss

Appendix C

IQ tests

An IQ test, if needed, is administered by a psychologist, to produce an IQ score. This is a statistical score compared to average intelligence which is 100, with 71 to 130 considered to be within the normal range.

An IQ of 70 is an international benchmark of having a learning disability, people with a mild learning disability have an IQ of 50 to 70; which is by far the largest group within the general population as estimates suggest a prevalence of around 25 per 1000 population (Department of Health 2001). Some individuals with mild learning disabilities may even not be identified because they function and adapt well socially. People with moderate learning disabilities have an IQ of 35 to 50; severe learning disabilities has meant an IQ of 20 to 35 and an IQ of less than 20 puts people in a category of having a profound learning disability. We describe this as the bell shaped distribution of intelligence.

Table 2 **Levels of learning disability**

Level of learning disability	Level of IQ	Level of social skills
Mild	50 to 69	<ul><li>Mental age 9-12 years</li><li>good understanding and use of language</li><li>full independence in self-care skills</li><li>some help required with reading and writing</li><li>fully mobile</li></ul>
Moderate	35 to 49	<ul><li>Mental age 6-9 years</li><li>limited language skills</li><li>supervision required with self-care</li><li>limited reading and writing skills</li><li>good mobility</li></ul>
Severe	20 to 34	<ul><li>Mental age 3-6 years</li><li>marked impairment of language and communication</li><li>constant supervision required</li><li>poor reading and writing skills</li><li>usually limited mobility</li></ul>
Profound	less than 20	<ul><li>Mental age <3 years</li><li>only basic understanding of communication</li><li>constant supervision required</li><li>no reading and writing skills</li><li>generally immobile</li></ul>

A level of IQ of over 70 is defined as being in the 'normal' IQ range; the average IQ for the general population being 100.

International diagnostic criteria still refer to a person's 'mental age' and in the past, people used to refer to people as having a particular mental age; by comparing a person's abilities to a chronological age. They would say 'John is 27 but he has a mental age of 4'. This is now seen as inaccurate and insulting to people with a learning disability, although very occasionally the press still describe people in this way.

There is considerable variation in levels of intellectual functioning among adults with Down syndrome. There are also differences in different areas of intellectual functioning, eg in reading, speech and number work. In the past, the average IQ levels for adults with Down syndrome were reported to be around 30-45, the lower end of so-called 'moderate impairment'. This level is no longer accurate. It is almost certain that as a result of better access to education and family support many adults with Down syndrome will score in the mild learning disability range and some in the 'normal' range.

Appendix D

Further reading and sources of information

Annual Health Checks for People with a Learning Disability. Royal College of General Practitioners. Download guides at http://bit.ly/18oC5N8 [Accessed 3.9.13]

Berg, J M, Karlinsky, H and Holland, A J (1993) *Alzheimer Disease, Down Syndrome, and their Relationship.* Oxford: Oxford Medical Publications

Bradley, A (2013) *Health and Safety for Learning Disability Workers.* Birmingham: BILD/Sage

Buckley, S and Sacks, B (1987) *The Adolescent with Down's Syndrome.* Portsmouth: Portsmouth Down's Syndrome Trust

Carr, J (1995) *Down's Syndrome, Children Growing Up.* Cambridge: Cambridge University Press

Chicoine, B and McGuire, D (2010) *Guide to Good Health: For Teens and Adults with Down Syndrome.* Bethesda, MD: Woodbine House

Corbett, J (2007) *Health Care Provision for People with Learning Disabilities: A Guide for Health Professionals.* Oxford: Wiley

Cuskelly, M, Jobling, A and Buckley, S (2002) *Down Syndrome Across the Life Span.* Oxford: Wiley

Dodd, K, Turk, V and Christmas, M (2009) *Down's Syndrome and Dementia: A Resource for Carers and Support Staff.* Second edition. Birmingham: BILD

Donaghy, V, Bernal, J, Tuffrey-Wijne, I and Hollins, S (2002) *Getting On With Cancer.* London: Books Beyond Words

Down Syndrome Healthcare Guidelines. National Down Syndrome Society. Download from http://bit.ly/15X63c9 [Accessed 3.9.13]

Down Syndrome Association of West Michigan (2010) *Guide for Parents of Teens and Young Adults with Down Syndrome.* Download from: http://bit.ly/1dJ8y6X [Accessed 3.9.13]

Down's Syndrome Association (2011) *Annual Health Checks for Adults with Down's Syndrome.* Download from: http://bit.ly/14m9gUt [Accessed 3.9.12]

Equal Access to Breast and Cervical Screening for Disabled Women (2006) Public Health England. Download from http://bit.ly/15xV37H [Accessed 3.9.13]

European Down Syndrome Association (no date) *Healthcare Guidelines for People with Down Syndrome.* Download from: http://bit.ly/1alebaO [Accessed 3.9.13]

FAIR (2010) *Keep Yourself Healthy: A Guide to Checking your Breasts*. NHS Health Scotland. Download from http://bit.ly/15Xd64x [Accessed 3.9.13]

Fiske, J, Dougall, A and Lewis, D (2009) *A Clinical Guide to Special Care Dentistry*. London: British Dental Association

Hearing Aids. Live Well, NHS Choices. Download from: http://bit.ly/14XEa3T [Accessed 3.9.13]

HFT Family Carer Support Service (2011) *Using the Mental Capacity Act. A Resource for Families and Friends of People with Learning Disabilities*. Download from: http://bit.ly/1dGj4f8 [Accessed 3.9.13]

HFT Family Carer Support Service offer a range of health resources:

- *Hospital Passport*
- *Working Together: Guidance for Hospitals, Families and Paid Support Staff*
- *Basic Personal Care MOT*
- *What do I need to know about NHS Continuing Healthcare?*
- *Good Healthcare for All – What Can I Expect from the NHS?*

Download these guides from: http://bit.ly/14Yd1xK [Accessed 3.9.13]

Hollins, S, Bernal J and Gregory, M (1996) *Going to the Doctor*. London: Books Beyond Words

Hollins, S, Bernal, J and Gregory, M (1998) *Going to Out-Patients*. London: Books Beyond Words

Hollins, S and Besser, R (2012) *Getting on with Type 1 Diabetes*. London: Books Beyond Words

Hollins, S, Besser, R and Dowling, L (2012) *Getting on with Type 2 Diabetes*. London: Books Beyond Words

Hollins, S, Blackman, N and Eley, R (2012) *Ann has Dementia*. London: Books Beyond Words

Hollins, S, Cappuccio, F and Adeline, P (2006) *Looking After My Heart*. London: Books Beyond Words

Hollins, S, Dowling, S and Blackman, N (2003) *When Somebody Dies*. London: Books Beyond Words

Hollins, S and Perez, W (2000) *Looking After My Breasts*. London: Books Beyond Words

Hollins, S, Perez, W and Abdelnoor, A (2000) *Keeping Healthy 'Down Below'*. London: Books Beyond Words

Hollins, S and Sireling, L (1989) *When Dad Died*. London: Books Beyond Words

Hollins, S and Sireling, L (1989) *When Mum Died*. London: Books Beyond Words

Hollins, S and Wilson, J (2004) *Looking After My Balls*. London: Books Beyond Words

Lott, L T and McCoy, EE (1992) *Down Syndrome – Advances in Medical Care*. New York: Wiley

McGuire, D and Chicoine, B (2006) *Mental Wellness in Adults with Down Syndrome: A Guide to Emotional and Behavioral Strengths and Challenges.* Bethesda, MD: Woodbine House

Nadel, L and Rosenthal, D (1995) *Down Syndrome. Living and Learning in the Community.* New York: Wiley

Newton, R (2004) *The Down's Syndrome Handbook: A Practical Guide for Parents and Carers.* London: Vermilion

Prasher, V P (2005) *Alzheimer's Disease and Dementia in Down Syndrome and Intellectual Disabilities.* Oxon: Radcliffe Publishing Ltd

Prasher, V P (2008) *Neuropsychological Assessments of Dementia in Down Syndrome and Intellectual Disabilities.* London: Springer-Verlag

Pueschel, S M and Rynders, J E (1982) *Down Syndrome. Advances in Biomedicine and the Behavioural Sciences.* Cambridge, Mass: Academic Guild Publishers

Pueschel, S, Tingley, C, Rynders, J, Crocker, A and Crutcher, D (1987) *New Perspectives on Down Syndrome.* MD: Brookes Publishing Co

Pueschel, S M and Pueschel, K (1992) *Biomedical Concerns in Persons with Down Syndrome.* MD: Brookes Publishing Co

Pueschel, S M (2006) *Adults with Down Syndrome.* Baltimore, MD: Brookes Publishing Co

Rondal, J A, Perera, J, Nadel, L and Comblain, A (1996) *Down's Syndrome. Psychological, Psychobiological and Socioeducational Perspectives.* Oxford: Wiley-Blackwell

Rondall, J, Rasore-Quartino, A and Soresi, S (2004) *The Adult with Down Syndrome: A New Challenge for Society.* Oxford: Wiley

Stratford, B and Gunn, P (eds)(1996) *New Approaches to Down Syndrome.* London: Continuum International Publishing Group Ltd

Legislation, policies and reports

Adults with Incapacity (Scotland) Act 2000 Download from: http://bit.ly/IH5jjf [Accessed 3.9.13]

Department for Constitutional Affairs (2007) *Mental Capacity Act 2005. Code of Practice*. Download from: http://bit.ly/1a5Qm3n [Accessed 3.9.13]

Department of Health (2001) *Valuing People. A New Strategy for Learning Disability for the 21st Century. A White Paper*. Download from: http://bit.ly/17DUyVN [Accessed 3.9.13]

Department of Health (2008) *Mental Capacity Act 2005. Deprivation of Liberty Safeguards*. Download from: http://bit.ly/1cF1R2x [Accessed 3.9.13]

Department of Health (2009) *Valuing People Now: A New Three-Year Strategy for People with Learning Disabilities*. Download from: http://bit.ly/1fywmHd [Accessed 3.9.13]

Department of Health (2013) *The NHS Constitution for England*. Download from: http://bit.ly/15y9Xea [Accessed 3.9.13]

DHSSPSNI (2005) *Equal Lives: Review of Policy and Services for People with a Learning Disability in Northern Ireland*. Download from: http://bit.ly/15XSVDI [Accessed 3.9.13]

Scottish Government (2012) *Your Health, Your Rights. The Charter of Patient Rights and Responsibilities*. Download from: http://bit.ly/1dOt0E8 [Accessed 3.9.13]

Scottish Government (2013) *The Keys to Life – Improving Quality of Life for People with Learning Disabilities*. Download from: http://bit.ly/17NBVm6 [Accessed 3.9.13]

Welsh Assembly Government (2007) *Statement on Policy and Practice for Adults with a Learning Disability*. Download from: http://bit.ly/15DbCrY [Accessed 3.9.13]

Appendix E

Details of organisations and websites for further information and advice

United Kingdom

Action on Hearing Loss
Experts in providing support for people with hearing loss and tinnitus.

www.actiononhearingloss.org.uk

Tel: 0808 808 0123

Alzheimer Scotland
Provides a wide range of specialist services for people with dementia and their carers.

www.alzscot.org

Tel: 0808 808 3000

Alzheimer's Society
Works to improve the quality of life of people affected by dementia in England, Wales and Northern Ireland.

www.alzheimers.org.uk

Tel: 0300 222 11 22

Ann Craft Trust – Acting Against Abuse
Works to ensure that organisations that support children and adults with learning disabilities are aware of abuse and protection issues.

www.anncrafttrust.org

Tel: 0115 951 5400

Bereavement and Learning Disabilities
Information on bereavement and learning disabilities with useful links and resources.

www.bereavementanddisability.org.uk

Tel: 01782 556653

British Dietetic Association
Aims to advance the science and promote training and education in the science and practice of dietetics and associated subjects.

www.bda.uk.com

Tel: 0121 200 8080

British Institute of Learning Disabilities (BILD)
Offer services that help develop organisations who provide services, and the people who give support, to help ensure that people are supported with dignity and respect and can make choices and decisions about their lives.

www.bild.org.uk

Tel: 0121 415 6960

Brook
Provides free and confidential sexual health services and advice for young people under 25.

www.brook.org.uk

Tel: 0808 802 1234

Carers UK
Offer support to help the millions of people who look after an older, disabled or seriously ill family member or friend.

www.carersuk.org

Tel: 0808 808 7777

Down's Heart Group
Offer support and information relating to heart conditions associated with Down's Syndrome.

www.dhg.org.uk

Tel: 0844 288 4800

Down's Syndrome Association
Providing information and support on all aspects of living with Down's syndrome to all who need it.

www.downs-syndrome.org.uk

Tel: 0333 1212 300

Down Syndrome Education International
Work with parents and teachers worldwide to improve educational outcomes for children with Down syndrome.

www.dseinternational.org

Tel: 0300 330 0750

Down Syndrome International
Committed to improving quality of life for people with Down syndrome worldwide and promoting their inherent right to be accepted and included as valued and equal members of their communities.

www.ds-int.org

Tel: 020 8614 5124

Down Syndrome Medical Interest Group (DSMIG)
Website provides essential information for health care professionals on 'best practice' medical care for people with Down syndrome in the UK and Ireland. Also includes a set of resources for parents and carers.

www.dsmig.org.uk

Down Syndrome Research and Practice Journal
This journal offers the best of Down syndrome research, practice, news and reviews in accessible formats for families, practitioners and researchers. All papers are available online for free from this website:

www.down-syndrome.org/research-practice

Down Syndrome Research
Charity with international links and a objective to improve the outcome for all people born with Trisomy 21 (T21) which is the cause of Down syndrome (DS), and the most common cause (at birth) of learning disability.

www.dsrf-uk.org

Down Syndrome Scotland
Work to help people with Down's syndrome reach their full potential by providing information, services and wsupport to them, their families, carers and professionals.

www.dsscotland.org.uk

Tel: 0131 313 4225

English Federation of Disability Sport
The national body for disabled people in sport and physical activity throughout England.

www.efds.co.uk

Tel 01509 227750

Family Planning Association
Educate and inform thousands of people about sexual health each year and campaign to improve sexual health services.

www.fpa.org.uk

Tel: 0845 122 6860 (UK)
Tel: 0845 122 8687 (N. Ireland)

Macmillan
Provide practical, medical and financial support and push for better cancer care.

www.macmillan.org.uk

Tel: 0808 808 0000

Mencap
Work in partnership with people with a learning disability, and all their services support people to live life as they choose.

www.mencap.org.uk

Tel: 0808 808 1111

Partially Sighted Society
Provides information, advice, training, equipment and clear print material for people with a visual impairment to help them to make the best use of their remaining sight.

http://partsight.org.uk

Tel: 0844 477 4966

Riding for the Disabled Association
Dedicated to improving the lives of thousands of people through education, therapy and fun.

www.rda.org.uk

Tel: 0845 658 1082

Royal National Institute of Blind People (RNIB)
Offers information, support and advice to almost two million people with sight loss.

www.rnib.org.uk

Tel: 0303 123 9999

The National Autistic Society
Provide information, support and pioneering services, and campaign for a better world for people with autism.

www.autism.org.uk

Tel: 020 7833 2299

UK Sports Association for People with Learning Disability
Encourage the development of sustainable, integrated quality sports provision for people with a learning disability.

www.uksportsassociation.org

Tel: 020 7490 3057

Understanding Intellectual Disability and Health
Web-based information for medical students and other health professionals

www.intellectualdisability.info

Europe

European Down Syndrome Association
Brings together organisations from across Europe, sharing information and promoting collaboration to improve life for people with Down syndrome and their families.

www.down-syndrome.eu

Ireland

Down's Syndrome Ireland
Dedicated to being the primary source of information and support to people with Down syndrome, their families and the professional community.

www.downsyndrome.ie

United States of America

Adult Down Syndrome Center
Enhancing the wellbeing of adolescents, 12 and older, and adults with Down syndrome using a team approach to provide comprehensive, holistic, community-based health care services.

www.advocatehealth.com/adultdown

National Down Syndrome Society
The national advocate for the value, acceptance and inclusion of people with Down syndrome.

www.ndss.org

National Down Syndrome Congress
Provide information, advocacy and support concerning all aspects of life for individuals with Down syndrome.

www.ndsccenter.org

Appendix F

Index

Added to a page number 'f' denotes a figure and 't' denotes a table.

abdomen, swollen   80, 81, 134
abdominal pain   77
   as a symptom of disease   60, 78, 79, 80, 81, 82, 84, 86, 87, 89, 98, 129, 134, 140
abnormal heart rate   53, 60, 68, 131
abscess   71, 117, 118
absences   105
accommodation (vision) abnormal   41
acne   119
acquired hypothyroidism   127
acrocyanosis   124
Action on Hearing Loss   34, 52
acute kidney failure   99, 100
acute lymphoblastic leukaemia (ALL)   133, 134
acute myeloid leukaemia (AML)   133, 134
adaptive behaviour   18
adaptive function   18
adaptive function tests   19
adenoids   150
   enlarged   67, 71
Adults with Incapacity Act (Scotland) (2000)   12
advocacy   12, 94
age
   blood pressure by   54f
   and obesity   23
   onset of dementia   141
   risk of Down syndrome   8
   and social competence   20
age-appropriate behaviours   18
ageing
   eye problems   38, 43
   hearing loss   48
   premature   20, 38, 46, 122, 135
   reduction in height   21
   vitamins supplementation   26
   see also older adults
aggression   45, 82, 143, 144, 145, 146

airway problems   64, 66, 70
allergies and allergic reactions   42, 43, 44, 65, 66, 67, 68, 70, 80, 120
alopecia   122
Alzheimer's disease   135, 141–2
amenorrhoea   87–8
anaemia   65, 131–2
   as a symptom of disease   53, 80, 81, 99, 127
anorexia   87, 99
anti-oxidants   26, 46, 142
anti-vascular endothelial growth factor   46
antibodies   81, 84, 127
anxiety, about visiting doctors   29
anxiety disorders   142–3, 146
   as a symptom of disease   137, 138, 139
aortic coarctation   58, 150
apathy   141, 145
aplastic anaemia   132
appetite
   disturbance   70, 84, 122, 128, 129, 138, 140
   reduction   24
arthritis
   osteoarthritis   113
   rheumatoid   114
   susceptibility to   24
assistive technology   34
asthma   64, 68, 82
astigmatism   40–1
atherosclerosis   62
athlete's foot   124
atlanto-axial instability (AAI)   102, 110–11
atlanto-occipital instability (AOI)   110–11
atonic seizures   105
atopic dermatitis   120–1
atrial septal defect (ASD)   58, 150
atrioventricular septal defect (AVSD)   58
attention deficit disorder (ADD)   147
audiologists   48, 52
audiology services   34
autistic spectrum conditions   75, 142, 145–6
autoimmune conditions   114, 122, 123, 127, 128, 132, 135
   see also immune system problems

backache 86, 87
bacterial infections 42, 65, 67, 69, 70, 120
bad breath 117
Barrett's oesophagus 82
behavioural change
　due to bereavement 138
　misdiagnosis in 40
　as a sign of abuse 95
　as a symptom of disease 39, 48, 49, 50, 71, 76, 77, 78, 79, 86, 87, 89, 90, 98, 99, 105, 110, 120, 128, 131, 140, 141, 143, 144, 145, 146, 147
behavioural programmes/therapy 24, 138, 140, 143, 144, 145, 147
benign prostatic hyperplasia 100
benign prostatic hypertrophy 100
bereavement 138–9, 141
'best interest' decisions 12
birth hypothyroidism 126
birth rate 8
bleeding, as a symptom of disease 134
blepharitis 42
bloating 79, 83, 86, 87
blood diseases 131–5
blood glucose levels 25, 129
blood pressure (BP) 54–6
　abnormal 55
　age and 54
　average 54
body mass index (BMI) 22, 23
boils 120
bone density 113
bone loss 90
bone marrow disease 131, 132
bowel disease
　bowel cancer 81
　irritable bowel syndrome 82
　as a symptom of disease 78, 79, 80
bowel obstruction 78–9
bradycardia 53
brain abscess 61
brain cancer 89
breast checks 93
breast screening 93
breast tenderness/discomfort 86, 87, 89

breathing problems
　due to heart lesions 58
　as a symptom of disease 53, 55, 56, 60, 61, 62, 74, 99, 128, 131, 138, 143
　see also respiratory problems
British Dietetic Association 33
bronchitis 64, 69
bruising 134
Bruxisim 118

calorie intake 23, 24, 25, 76
cancers see individual diseases
Candida albicans 90
candida infection (Candidiasis)
　in men 92
　in women 90
carbohydrate deficiency 25
cardiovascular disease 94
care in the community 9
care managers 31–2
carer support 143
　see also short break services
caries (tooth decay) 115, 116, 118
cataracts 43, 129
cerumen 48, 50
cervical smear tests 93
Charter of Patients' Rights and Responsibilities 29
check-ups 10, 11, 27, 28, 40, 41, 93, 115, 151
chelitis 123
chest infections 58, 60, 61, 64, 68, 71
chest pain 53, 61, 62, 71
choking 71, 74, 105, 143
cholesterol 62
chronic prostatitis 101
circulatory problems 53–6, 129, 132
cochlear implants 49
Coeliac disease 80–1
colds 50, 64–5
coma 103, 104, 129
communication, and hearing loss 49, 52
community learning disability nurses 31
community learning disability team (CLDT) 31, 32

Index　　165

community paediatric services 30
complaints procedures 29
concentration problems 71, 138, 140
concussion 103
conductive hearing loss 48, 50
confusion 55, 56, 71, 128, 129
congestive heart failure 59
conjunctivitis 42–3
consciousness
   loss of 103–4, 128
   see also fainting
consent
   informed 95
   resources about 29
constipation 75, 76, 79
   as a symptom of disease 75, 77, 78, 82, 89, 127
continuous positive airway pressure 72
contraception 93–4
   barrier methods 94, 106
   Depo-Provera 94
   intrauterine devices 94
   oral contraceptive pill 86, 87, 88, 94
corneal protrusion 44
corneal reflection 41
corneal swelling 44
coronary artery disease 62
cough 64
   as a symptom of disease 60, 67, 68, 69, 70, 71, 82, 103
cutis marmorata 124
cyanosis 59, 61, 68, 69
cystitis 98
cysts 89, 117, 119

day centres 35
dehydration 55, 70, 75, 80
delirium 139
delusions 140, 141, 144, 145
dementia 20, 131, 137, 141–2
   hypothyroidism and 127
   misdiagnosis 40, 48
   susceptibility to 28
dental care 115, 116
   heart problems 60, 61
   mouth ulcers 78
   support services 35
   see also teeth

dentists
   community 35
   specialists in learning disability 35
depression 70, 140, 143
   disorders due to 79, 87, 137, 141
   due to bereavement 138
   misdiagnosis 40, 48
   as a sign of abuse 95
   susceptibility to 28
   as a symptom of disease 75
diabetes 120, 128–9
   disorders due to 92, 99
   susceptibility to 24
   as a symptom of disease 62, 76
   Type 1 128, 129
   Type 2 128, 129
diabetic ketoacidosis 128, 129
diarrhoea 80
   as a symptom of disease 79, 80, 81, 82, 87, 89, 128, 143
diastolic blood pressure 54
diet 79
   balanced 21, 26
   control of disease 81, 83, 86, 106, 113
   and obesity 23, 24, 26
   variety in 27
   see also healthy eating; nutrition
dietary supplements 26
dieticians 27, 33, 75, 76
dieting 24, 27
digestive problems 24, 73–84
digestive system 73f
dislocation of joints 109
dizziness 55, 56, 129, 131, 143
doctors, anxiety about visiting 29
Down syndrome
   information sources 156–9
   life-expectancy 8
   numbers diagnosed during pregnancy 8
   organisations 35, 36, 160–3
   population 8
   risk factors 8
drug therapy
   disorders due to 25, 53, 55, 65, 78, 80, 88, 104, 113, 127, 133
   weight reduction 25
   see also individual disorders
dysmenorrhoea 87, 94
dysphagia 75

ear   47
ear infections   50–1, 64, 67, 74, 102
ear plugs   51
earache   49, 50, 66
early intervention   19
earwax   48, 50
Easy Read books   29
eating
    learning good habits   27
    see also healthy eating; over-eating
eating problems   75–6
    as a symptom of disease   115, 146
echocardiography   53, 57, 59, 60
eczema   120–1
education, access to   18
Eisenmenger complex   61
emollients   121
emotional problems   137–47
    disorders due to   23, 68, 74, 75, 77, 80, 82, 86, 121
    as a sign of abuse   95
    as a symptom of disease   39, 48, 49, 50, 77, 78, 87, 98, 99, 105, 110, 120, 131, 140, 145
encephalitis   70
endocarditis   60–1, 115, 117
endometriosis   89
enzyme levels, low   25
epilepsy   25, 79, 86, 104–5
    identification cards   106
    see also seizures
epistaxis   65
esotropia   41
Eustachian tube   51, 150
exercise
    benefits of   24, 76, 79, 112
    risks of   53, 62
exotropia   41
external ear infections   50
eye(s)
    as indicators of Down syndrome   38
    parts of   39f
eye pain   44
eye rubbing   42, 43, 44
eye specialists   38, 44
eyelids, inflammation of   42
eyestrain   39, 40, 41, 102

fainting   103–4
    as a symptom of disease   53, 56, 60, 61, 62, 87, 131
family meals   27
family members
    education about epilepsy   106
    role of   11–12, 73
    support from   49
fatigue   58
    as a symptom of disease   59, 60, 61, 62, 64, 70, 80, 81, 86, 87, 127, 131, 132, 134, 138, 140
feet problems   112
    athlete's foot   124
fever   50, 53, 59, 60, 65, 66, 69, 70, 80, 84, 98, 102, 104, 120, 133, 134, 139
fish oils   87
floaters   45
fluid retention   86, 99
folate deficiency   25, 135
folic acid deficiency   131
follicle stimulating hormone (FSH)   90
friendships   19

gallstones   24, 82
gastroesophageal reflux disease (GORD)   82–3
gender
    and obesity   23
    prevalence of Down syndrome   8
    and stature   21
general practitioners (GP)   10, 30
    resources for   29
generalised seizures   105
genetic testing   141
genitourinary care   85
gingivitis   117
gland disorders   55, 67, 87, 100, 127, 128, 134
glands   125, 126f
glaucoma   40, 44, 102
glucose metabolism, impaired   25
glue ear   48, 50, 51, 67
gluten allergy   80
gluten-free diet   81
Going to the Doctor   29
gout   130, 132

Index   167

Grave's disease   127
grommets   51, 150
growth   21
   charts   21
   delayed   21
growth hormone   23, 130
growth hormone therapy   21
gums, inflammation of   117–18
gynaecological problems   77, 86

H. pylori   83
haemodialysis   100
haemoglobin   131, 132
hair problems   119, 120
   hair loss   122, 127
halitosis   117
hallucinations   138, 139, 140, 141, 144, 145
Hashimoto's Thyroiditis   127
hayfever   66–7
   see also rhinitis
head posture, abnormal   45
head rests   111
head trauma   103
headache   94, 102
   as a symptom of disease   39, 40,
      41, 55, 56, 61, 64, 66, 67, 69, 70,
      86, 87, 89, 131, 132, 140
health action plans   10–11
health care   9
   access to   10
   levels of support   12–15
   provision   10–12
   role of family members and
      paid staff   11–12
   targeting   9
health decisions   10, 12
health passports   11
health professionals   28, 29, 30–3
health promotion
   access to   24
   sexual   85, 93
healthy eating   26
   guidelines   27
   information and advice   27
   see also diet; nutrition

hearing aids   48, 49, 51–2
   services   34
   therapists   52
hearing impairment   47–52
   support services   34
   susceptibility to   9
   as a symptom of disease   127
   tests   48
hearing loss   48, 50, 51
   conductive   48, 50
   information and advice   52
   sensorineural   48, 49
heart, structure   56, 57f
heart lesions   58, 59, 61
   aortic coarctation   58, 150
   atrial septal defect (ASD)   58
   mitral valve prolapse (MVP)   59
   patent ductus arteriosus   58, 150
   tetralogy of Fallot   58, 59
   ventricular septal defect (VSD)   58, 59, 150
heart murmurs   59, 60
heart problems   19, 53, 55, 56–62, 129, 133
   heart failure   54, 56, 59–60, 61,
      69, 72, 127, 131
   hole in the heart   56
   susceptibility to   9, 24
heart rate   53, 54, 60, 68, 131
height   21, 22f
Heimlich Manoeuvre   74
Hepatitis A   84
Hepatitis B   84, 135
   immunisation   136
Hepatitis C   84
high blood pressure see hypertension
HIV virus   95
holistic approach   18
hormonal treatment   86, 89, 107, 119, 138
hormone problems   23, 125–30
hormone replacement therapy (HRT)
   90, 113, 130
hormones   125
hospital passports   11
hyperactivity   138, 143
hyperkinetic disorder   147
hypermetropia   40
hypertension   24, 25, 55, 72, 90, 94, 99, 129, 132
   see also blood pressure

hyperthyroidism   53, 76, 80, 125, 127–8
hypertropia   41
hypoglycaemia   129, 143
hypomania   144
hypospadias   91
hypotension   54, 55–6, 103
hypothermia   53
hypothyroidism   23, 24, 27, 53, 79, 87, 125, 126–7, 128, 141
hypotropia   41
hypoxia   61

illusions   139
immune function, vitamins and improved   26
immune system problems   135–6
    see also autoimmune conditions
immunisations   135–6
independence   18, 19, 38
infection
    disorders due to   78, 80, 87, 88, 99, 121, 124, 132
    as a symptom of disease   98, 128, 132, 133, 134
    see also individual types
influenza   50, 70
    immunisation   136
informed consent   95
inhalers   68
insulin   23, 128, 129
intellectual development   18–20
intellectual functioning   18–19
    vitamins and   26
intelligent quotient (IQ)   18, 19, 150
    tests   18, 19, 154–5
internet   36
iodine deficiency   127
iron replacement   88
iron tablets   127, 132
irradiation   83
irritability   71, 80, 81, 82, 87, 95, 102, 128, 138, 143, 144
irritable bowel syndrome (IBS)   82

jaundice   84
joint aspiration   110
joint problems
    degeneration   113
    dislocation   109
    painful   110
    as a symptom of disease   130, 134

keratoconus   40, 44, 59
kidney problems   55, 61, 91, 97, 98, 99, 129
    kidney failure   55, 99–100, 101, 103

lactose intolerance   81
lazy eye   41, 42
learning disabilities
    level of   154t
    social competence   20
legs, swollen   60, 61, 62, 63
leukaemia   132, 133–4
Lewy-body dementia   141
life-expectancy   8, 142
lifelong learning   20
light intolerance   44
lip problems   59, 61, 68, 123
liver
    disease   60, 84, 94
    enlarged   60, 134
    failure   84
    inflammation   84
long-sightedness   40
low blood pressure see hypotension
lung(s)
    collapsed   68, 71
    disease   24, 56, 57, 59, 72
    fluid in   60
    inflammation   70, 71, 75

macrocytosis   135
macular degeneration   46
malabsorption syndrome   80–1
malnutrition   77
malocclusions   116
mania   144
maxillomandibular advancement   72
medical checklist   151–3
medical model   18

Index   169

medical problems
    susceptibility to 9
    see also individual disorders
medication *see* drug therapy
megavitamin therapy 26, 76
memory impairment 9, 138, 140, 141
menhorrhagia 88
meningitis 70, 102
menopause 87, 89–90, 113
    oestrogen replacement therapy 113
menstruation 86, 89
    see also periods
mental capacity, decision-making 12
Mental Capacity Act (2005) 12
mental health problems 70, 137–47
    as a symptom of disease 127
metabolic disturbances 77
metabolism 23
middle ear infection 50, 70
migraine headaches 102, 103
mini pill 88
mitral valve prolapse (MVP) 59
mood swings 86, 89, 90, 139, 144, 145
mouth ulcers 78, 115, 134
multi-professional community paediatric services 30
muscle wasting 77
myelofibrosis 134
myoclonic seizures 104, 105
myoclonus 106–7
myopia 39–40

nail problems 112, 121, 124
nasal discharge 64, 67, 68
nausea 78, 84, 87, 94, 99, 129
nervous system problems 25, 102–8
neutropenia 133, 135
NHS Constitution 29
NHS system 30
non-Hodgkin's lymphoma 89
nosebleed 65
nutrition 21, 25
nutritional deficiency 25, 76, 78, 123
nutritional disorders 25

nutritional excess 25
nutritional supplementation 19, 26
nystagmus 45

obesity 19, 22–4
    diet and 23, 24, 26
    disorders due to 71, 82, 90
    levels of 22, 23
    measuring 22
    surgery for 24
    susceptibility to 9, 28
    as a symptom of disease 62
obsessive compulsive disorder (OCD) 28, 143–4
obstructive sleep apnoea 24, 67, 71–2
occupational therapists 32
oesophageal tears 75
older adults 9, 20, 70, 139, 141
    see also ageing
oligomenorrhoea 88
onchomycosis 124
ophthalmologist/optometrist 34, 38, 39, 43, 44
osteoarthritis 113
osteoporosis 90, 113
otitis externa 50
otitis media 50, 70
ovarian cancer 89, 94
over-eating 74, 77, 82
overweight 22, 23, 24, 26, 28
    see also obesity
ovulation 87

paediatricians 30–1
pallor 60, 75, 129, 131, 134
palpitations 53, 58, 89, 128, 143
panic attacks 142, 143
paranoia 145
partial seizures 105
Partially Sighted Society 35
patent ductus arteriosus 58, 150
pelvic examinations 86
peptic ulcer disease 83
perennial rhinitis 67
periodontitis 117–18

periods
   abnormal   127
   absence of   87–8
   cessation of   140
   early onset or delayed   85
   heavy   88, 89
   irregular   88
   painful   85, 87, 94
peripheral vascular disease   55
peritonitis   78
pernicious anaemia   131
person-centred approach   18
personal skills   20
personality change   141, 145
pharmacists   33
pharyngitis   65–6
phimosis   91
phobias   143, 146
physical activity   23, 40, 79, 101, 109
physiotherapists   32
plaques (dental)   116, 117
pleurisy   71
pneumonia   69, 70, 70–1
polycythaemia   60, 61, 132–3, 150
post-infection depression   70
posture, abnormal   45, 112, 141
pregnancy
   disorders due to   74, 87
   monitoring   130
   numbers diagnosed during   8
   sterilisation and   95
premature ageing   20, 38, 46, 122, 135
premenstrual syndrome (tension) (PMS)   86
presbycusis   48
progesteron   88
prostate cancer   100, 101
prostate enlargement   100–2
protein deficiency   25
psoralen and ultraviolet A light (PUVA)   123
psoriasis   121
psychiatrists   31
psychological problems   75, 137–47
psychological support   106, 112
psychological tests   18
psychologists   33, 75, 76

puberty   119, 127, 887
pulse rate, abnormal   53, 127

quality of life   9, 20, 38, 52

recovery position   104
recurrent headaches   102
recurrent seizures   104
red blood cells   131, 132, 135
refeeding syndrome   77
rehabilitation   107, 145
relationships   19
   difficulties with   147
   loss of close   138
resources   29
respiratory problems   64–72
   stepwise approach   68–9
   see also breathing problems
restless leg syndrome   108
restlessness   80, 139
retinal detachment   45
rheumatoid arthritis   114
rheumatoid factor   114
rhinitis   66–7
   perennial   67
   seasonal   66–7
   see also hayfever
rights-based approach   18
Royal National Institute of Blind People (RNI)   35
runny nose   66, 67

salt intake   25, 55, 56, 63
schizophrenia   145
scoliosis   112
seasonal rhinitis   66–7
seborrhoeic dermatitis   121–2
secondary generalised seizures   105
seizures   94, 103
   as a symptom of disease   80, 81
   see also epilepsy
selective hearing   48
selenium   26
self-care skills   18, 19, 20
   loss of   20, 140, 141, 145

self-harm 45, 95, 138, 140, 145
self-help groups 24
sensorineural hearing loss 48, 49
sensory impairment 28, 66, 67
septicaemia 71, 98
serous otitis 50
sex hormones 130
sexual abuse 95–6
    protection from 95
sexual health 85–96
    information and advice 94
    men 91–2
    promotion 93
    women 85–90
sexually transmitted diseases 95
short break services 35
short-sightedness 39–40
single seizures 104
sinusitis 64, 66, 67–8, 70, 102
skeletal problems 109
skin problems 119–24
    discolourization 59, 61, 63, 84, 124
    susceptibility to 9
    as a symptom of disease 60, 127, 128, 132
sleep apnoea 24, 67, 71–2, 82, 138
sleep disturbance 137–8
    as a symptom of disease 49, 71, 89, 140, 144
smell, loss of 66, 67
snoring 67, 71, 138
social competence 19–20
social development 18–20
social model 18
social services teams 32
social skills 18, 19
    decline in 140
    level of 154*t*
social workers 31–2
sore throat 65–6
    as a symptom of disease 70, 82
spacer device 69
speech and language therapists 32, 49, 52, 75
spots (acne) 119
squint 40, 41–2

stature 21
    average 22
status asthmaticus 68
status epilepticus 105
sterilisation 94–5
stools
    abnormal 79, 80, 83, 84
    blood in 73, 80, 83
strabismus (squint) 40, 41–2
stroke(s) 24, 55, 72, 102, 107, 133
support services 34–6
    for dementia 142
    internet 36
    sexual abuse 95
    voluntary 145
sweating 60, 66, 75, 89, 129, 143
systolic blood pressure 54

T tubes 51
tachycardia 53
teeth 114
    disease 115
    grinding 118
    malocclusions 116
    tooth decay 82, 115, 116, 118
    toothache 78, 102, 115, 116, 117
    see also dental care
testicles
    checks 93
    undescended 92
testicular cancer 92, 93
tetralogy of Fallot 58, 59
thirst 128
thrombosis 94
Thrush *see* candida infection
thyroid deficiency 135
thyroid disorders 53, 59, 125
    disorders due to 88, 123
    hyperthyroidism 53, 76, 80, 125, 127–8
    hypothyroidism 23, 24, 27, 53, 79, 87, 125, 126–7, 128, 141
    susceptibility to 9, 24, 28
thyroid gland 125
thyroid stimulating hormone (TSH) 125, 127, 128, 150
thyroxine hormone 125, 126, 127, 128, 150
tinea pedis 124

tiredness *see* fatigue
tonic-clonic seizures 104, 105
tonsillitis 66
transfer of medical care from child to adult services 30–1
transient ischaemic attack (TIA) 107
transient myeloproliferative disorder 135
treatment
    concerns about 29
    see also individual disorders
trembling 143
tremor 128
tri-iodothyronine 125
trichotillomania 122

unconsciousness 103–4
upper spine 110, 111f
uric acid levels 25, 110, 130
urinary problems 97–101
    as a symptom of disease 89, 90, 91, 100
    urinary tract infection 60, 74, 91, 98
    urinary tract obstruction 99
urinary system 97f

valve defects (heart) 56
varicose veins 63
vascular dementia 141
ventricular septal defect (VSD) 58, 59, 150
videotaping 71, 105
viral infections 42, 64, 70, 84, 90, 123, 133
visual impairment 38–46, 55
    screening for 38
    services for 34–5
    susceptibility to 9
    as a symptom of disease 102, 128, 132
    visual aids 40, 44
vitamins
    deficiency 131, 135, 141
    excessive intake 25
    supplementation 26, 46, 49, 65, 76, 81, 86, 87, 113, 120, 132
    Vitamin A 46
    Vitamin B1 87
    Vitamin B7 131
    Vitamin B12 132, 135
    Vitamin C 46, 49, 65, 120
    Vitamin D 81, 113
    vitamin E 26, 46, 86, 142

vitiligo 123
voluntary organisations 36
vomiting 74–5
    as a symptom of disease 78, 80, 84, 87, 99, 102, 129

weakness 56, 60, 71, 107, 109, 110, 129
Wechsler Adult Intelligence Scale 18
weight
    desirable 23
    keeping to a healthy 27
    see also obesity; overweight
weight gain
    due to medication 122
    as a symptom of disease 60, 86, 127, 140
    through dramatic weight loss 24
weight loss 76–7, 110
    principles 24
    as a symptom of disease 60, 76, 80, 128, 140
white blood cells 133

xerosis 122

zinc levels 25
zinc supplement 46, 120